Second edition

Hysterectomy

New

options

and

advances

Lorraine Dennerstein

Carl Wood

Ann Westmore

Melbourne

OXFORD UNIVERSITY PRESS

Oxford   Auckland   New York

OXFORD UNIVERSITY PRESS AUSTRALIA

Oxford   New York
Athens   Auckland   Bangkok   Bombay
Calcutta   Cape Town   Dar es Salaam   Delhi
Florence   Hong Kong   Istanbul   Karachi
Kuala Lumpur   Madras   Madrid   Melbourne
Mexico City   Nairobi   Paris   Singapore
Taipei   Tokyo   Toronto

and associated companies in
Berlin   Ibadan

OXFORD is a trade mark of Oxford University Press

National Library of Australia
Cataloguing-in-Publication data:

Dennerstein, Lorraine
   Hysterectomy: new options and advances

   2nd ed.
   Bibliography.
   Includes index.
   ISBN 0 19 553670 3.

   1. Hysterectomy. I. Wood, Carl, 1929–   . II. Westmore,
   Ann, 1953–   . III. Title.

618.1453

Cover photograph: International Photographic Library
Illustrations by Levent Efe
Text designed by R. T. J. Klinkhamer
Typeset by Desktop Concepts P/L, Melbourne
Printed by Australian Print Group
Published by Oxford University Press,
253 Normanby Road, South Melbourne, Australia

Contents

Preface

In the mid-1970s two of us (L.D. and C.W.) surveyed a group of women who had undergone hysterectomy some years earlier. The results dismayed and appalled us.

It was apparent, for example, that unfounded fears and incorrect information had contributed to a deterioration in the sexual relationships of many of those interviewed. Negative expectations became self-fulfilling, and a great deal of unnecessary suffering resulted.

Some of those women asked that we make the results available to the wider community. The upshot was *Hysterectomy: How to deal with the physical and emotional aspects*. The book was published by Oxford University Press in 1982 with a third author, the internationally recognised psychiatrist, Graham Burrows. It was reviewed widely and reached a large audience.

As the mid-1990s approached, however, it was clear that a complete update was needed. The visit to Melbourne in late 1993 of highly regarded North American gynaecologist, Dr Karen Carlson, gave the authors an opportunity to discuss the results of the Maine Women's Health Study in the context of the US experience of hysterectomy and non-surgical alternatives to it, and to assess these results in the light of findings from the Melbourne Women's Midlife Health Project. There was clearly an urgent need to acquaint women with information about the expanding range of options becoming available to them.

This book reflects the commitment of the authors to provide information directly to women in an accessible manner. It acknowledges the right of individuals to decide what will happen to their bodies during medical treatment, and to be fully informed about possible and likely outcomes of this treatment.

Lorraine Dennerstein
Carl Wood
Ann Westmore

Acknowledgments

Carl Wood thanks his wife Marie for her support, and Ann Westmore acknowledges the support of her family and friends. Thanks are also due to the many women whose case histories are recorded in this book. Their names have been changed to protect their privacy.

Abbreviations

The authors have compiled a list of abbreviations to promote good communication between readers and their medical advisers. This book uses plain English and explains relevant technical terms as they arise.

CIN	cervical intraepithelial neoplasia
D and C	dilatation and curettage
GnRH agonists	gonadotrophin-releasing hormone analogues
HPV	human papilloma virus
HRT	hormone replacement therapy (also referred to as hormone therapy)
LHRH agonists	luteinising hormone releasing hormone agonists
MRI	magnetic resonance imaging
NSAID	nonsteroidal anti-inflammatory drug
Pap test	Papanicolaou (cervical) smear test
PID	pelvic inflammatory disease
PMS	premenstrual syndrome

Introduction

The decision whether to have a hysterectomy, try some other treatment, or postpone any intervention and let nature take its course, is of great importance to many women. Hysterectomy is the surgical removal of the uterus, sometimes accompanied by oophorectomy, the removal of the ovaries. Most hysterectomies and oophorectomies performed these days are elective — meaning they are carried out by choice rather than as emergency or lifesaving procedures.

Hysterectomy is one of the most common major surgical procedures performed on women worldwide. In the United States alone, around 600 000 women have the operation each year. Yet many questions remain unanswered about the appropriateness of hysterectomy for those women having it, and its effects on health, sexuality and life expectancy.

The purpose of this book is not to advocate more or fewer operations, but to provide accurate, accessible and up-to-date information about it and about other options that may be worth considering. For there is strong evidence that individuals who are well informed about their situation and who take an active role in deciding what to do about it fare better than those who rely on other people to make important health decisions for them. It is hoped that this book will aid you in discussions with others whose lives are intimately affected by hysterectomy, as well as with doctors and other health carers whose views may be considered when making decisions about this and other options.

one

The uterus

The uterus is situated deep within the pelvis (figure 1). It makes its presence felt during the reproductive years, when its inner lining bleeds intermittently and its lower portion, the cervix, produces mucus secretions. During a woman's fertile years the uterus is the most prominent of the female reproductive organs, drawing attention with activities like menstruation and pregnancy. In contrast, before a girl reaches puberty and after a woman has her menopause, it moves through phases of change slowly and unobtrusively.

Position in the pelvis

Some women can accurately locate the position of their uterus because of the contractions they feel during orgasm or menstruation. These uterine contractions can be like pleasant ripples and are an enjoyable part of sex for some, while other women find them painful. For women who don't experience these clues, it can be helpful to picture where the uterus sits inside the abdomen: the vagina is below, the bladder in front, the loops of the bowel above, and the rectum behind (figure 2).

Figure 1   Two views of the female reproductive organs

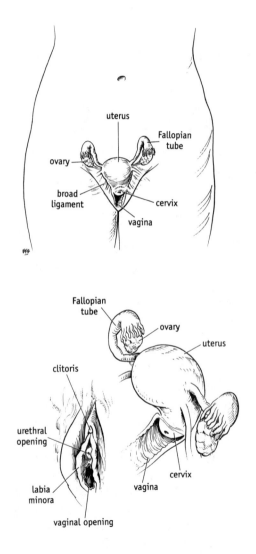

Figure 2   Cross-section of the body showing the position of the pelvic organs before and after hysterectomy

a Before hysterectomy

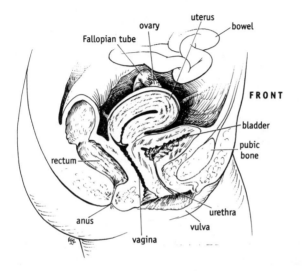

b After hysterectomy

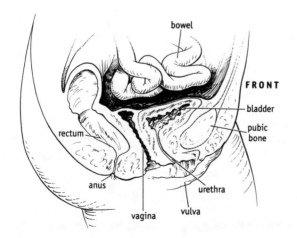

Strong support tissues called ligaments hold the uterus in place in the pelvis. If these ligaments are not able to provide the necessary support and the uterus becomes displaced (this is one type of prolapse, see chapter 2), this can create pain or changed function in the four surrounding organs. For example, pain during sex may result from the uterus pressing on and even into the vagina, while pressure on the bladder from the uterus can lead to urinary incontinence.

Appearance and function

The uterus is about the size and shape of a small hollow pear with its wide end upwards. Two fine tubes, the Fallopian tubes, branch outwards from the upper part of the uterus towards the ovaries. During reproductive life, a mature egg bursts from an ovary at approximately monthly intervals. In the normal course of events, an egg travels through a Fallopian tube to the uterus. On the way there, conception can occur if the egg meets and fuses with a sperm cell. The resulting embryo may develop into a viable pregnancy if it successfully embeds in the uterus.

The largest part of the uterus, the myometrium, is strong and flexible, being composed of thick bands of muscle and elastic tissue that run in several directions. This muscular web enables the uterus to be either small and tidy, somewhat like a clenched fist or, should conception occur, to stretch and grow into a strong, flexible capsule capable of nourishing and protecting a developing baby. The lower end of the uterus, the cervix, has some specialised functions including the production of lubricative or dense secretions at different times of the menstrual cycle. These secretions help minimise friction during sexual intercourse and seem to have a role in sperm movement through the vagina and cervix. During the Pap or cervical smear test, the cervix is the tissue that is sampled.

In addition to the thick myometrium and the cervix, the other important component of the uterus is its very active inner lining, called the endometrium. This is shed during menstruation or, if circumstances permit and a pregnancy occurs, it provides nutrients to an embryo. Before a girl has her first period (an event referred to as the menarche) and after a woman has her last (menopause), the endometrium usually consists of a thin layer of cells which may grow and be shed slowly without any menstrual bleeding.

The fertile years see a big change with menstruation typically occurring for several days about once every month. In the lead up to the menstrual bleed, row upon row of endometrial cells grow rapidly, influenced by sex hormones from the ovaries (particularly oestrogen and progesterone). Recent research suggests that the shedding process requires substances produced by the endometrium itself (such as the hormone-like prostaglandins and enzymes known as matrix metalloproteinases), together with decreasing levels of sex hormones.[1]

Some of the mechanisms of heavy, uncontrolled bleeding are not understood. Gaining insights into this phenomenon is obviously vital if improved ways to alleviate it are ever to be developed. A small protein called endothelin, discovered in the late 1980s, has been found to cause constriction of blood vessels in many parts of the body, and may be responsible for eventually ending any episode of blood loss. Recent research has revealed high levels of this protein in the endometrium around the time that the menstrual bleed comes to an end.[2]

While this research has been going on, the uterus has attracted increasing attention at a more general level. It has long been regarded by many people as a safe haven for a developing baby during pregnancy, but an unqualified nuisance thereafter. A 1987 editorial in the prestigious British medical journal *Lancet* expressed this view when it said:

> for the woman who is not interested in having children, or whose family is complete, this solution [hysterectomy] is often attractive ... [it promises] relief from her symptoms and other expected benefits — greater reliability at work, availability at all times for sexual intercourse, saving on sanitary protection, freedom from pregnancy and freedom from uterine cancer.[3]

Today, views such as this are being scrutinised due to a growing body of evidence which suggests that the uterus and cervix play an important part in sexual satisfaction for some women and men.[4] For perhaps as many as one in three women, contractions of the uterus contribute significantly to their experience of orgasm. As noted earlier, in pre-menopausal women the cervix also produces lubricative mucus for some days each menstrual cycle. This mucus, which is apparent in the days before ovulation, may be associated with increased interest in sex and less friction during intercourse. In addition, some men and women find that the tapping of the penis on the cervix during intercourse contributes to the pleasurable sensations they experience.

The uterus also seems to have psychological importance for some women, being associated with self-images of femininity and sexual attractiveness. This may be especially relevant in cultures where women's reproductive functions are highly valued. There is also a perception among some women that their partners treat them differently (find them less sexually attractive) after hysterectomy, suggesting that some men's notions of womanhood are closely allied to the presence of the uterus.

It is still the case — and this is controversial — that many surgeons remove both ovaries along with the uterus during hysterectomy procedures when there is no apparent ovarian disease or disorder. What's more, some women believe that they have not been consulted about this in advance. The reason typically given is prevention of ovarian cancer, which affects about one in seventy women, mostly over the age of sixty. Ovarian cancer is diagnosed in about 900 Australian women each year and about 550 die from it. The symptoms of pain, bleeding and swelling are usually not obvious until the disease has progressed to an advanced stage.

It is hoped that research findings indicating a role for the ovaries in women's long-term health will cause a reappraisal of this practice, especially as the risk for developing ovarian cancer in retained ovaries after hysterectomy is only about two in every 1000 women.[5] The available evidence indicates that even post-menopausal ovaries make sex hormones. These may be of value to women's health, particularly in helping maintain sexual interest and responsiveness, and bone strength. However the clinical evidence is inconclusive. It is clear that the long-term effect of removing the ovaries along with the uterus in the pre-menopausal years is to increase a woman's risk of heart disease — perhaps to three times that of non-hysterectomised women.[6] Furthermore, other research suggests that removal of both ovaries and the uterus increases the risk of osteoporosis, with increased loss of bone density and a higher incidence of fractures.[7]

Some studies indicate that even when women's ovaries are retained during hysterectomy there are likely to be some adverse impacts on blood fat levels and bone metabolism, although these changes are less marked than when both ovaries are removed. While the increased risks of heart disease and osteoporosis may be reversed by the careful use of hormone therapy (sometimes referred to as hormone replacement therapy or HRT), some women wonder about the merits of a surgical approach to their problems that will probably require the taking of hormone medications on a regular basis, with all that this entails. Even before a woman starts on hormone therapy, experienced clinicians advise *all* of the following:[8]

- a full check of general health, including the occurrence of any symptoms that may be related to menopause (such as hot flushes, headaches and vaginal dryness), and an assessment of any social and psychological factors that may contribute to symptoms
- a discussion of pre-hysterectomy menstrual cycles
- an assessment of lifestyle, including exercise and nutrition, patterns and use of medications, alcohol and cigarettes
- details of any previous medical, obstetric, gynaecological or psychological symptoms, and any personal or family history of breast cancer or breast lumps, blood clot formation, heart attack or stroke, fractures or osteoporosis, uterine fibroids, endometriosis, problems experienced with the Pill, liver disease, and any experience of premenstrual symptoms
- weight and blood pressure measurements, an examination of the breasts and vagina, and a Pap smear if the cervix remains

- a mammogram, especially if there is a family or personal history of breast problems
- an assessment of blood fat levels (cholesterol and triglycerides) if this has not been made during the previous twelve months
- a bone density scan if, at any time during the fertile years, menstruation stopped unexpectedly for longer than six months; and also if steroids are in use or have been used (for example, in asthma or thyroid treatment), if a recent fracture has occurred, or if there is a family history of fractures or osteoporosis.

After starting on hormone therapy, it usually takes six months for adverse effects to settle. These may include breast tenderness, fluid retention, nausea, weight gain or skin reactions. Medical check-ups two months after starting on hormones and then three months later are recommended. Once-yearly check-ups are advisable from then on, unless side-effects or other concerns occur, in which case prompt investigation is in order. During these check-ups, doctors should examine the breasts and arrange for a mammogram if this is overdue. When a woman decides to come off hormone therapy, the hormone dose should be reduced gradually rather than stopped suddenly.

A recent report by the Melbourne Women's Midlife Health Project suggests that the practice of removing ovaries during hysterectomies is not about to disappear.[9] The project is being undertaken by the Key Centre for Women's Health in Society at the University of Melbourne. Of 420 Melbourne women who had undergone a hysterectomy by the age of fifty-five years, only 59% had both ovaries intact, 21% had one ovary removed and a further 20% had both out. Four out of five women without ovaries or with one ovary had had them removed at the time of hysterectomy. There was no evidence of any trend towards conservation of ovaries during the previous twenty years.

The ovaries of a woman, whatever her age, should be retained during a hysterectomy unless their conservation is likely to jeopardise her health. The most common reasons for their removal are gynaecological disease such as endometriosis, recurrent ovarian cysts or ovarian adhesions that cause pain; an increased risk of ovarian or breast cancer; or a woman's preference.

Mind and body in uterine function

Links between reproductive function, mood and behaviour have been proposed for many years. Mothers who experience severe and persistent anxiety and depression after giving birth have been described as having postpartum depression. Women who consistently experience symptoms such as irritability, anxiety, aggression, depression and loss of concentration during the two weeks between ovulation and menstruation may be diagnosed as having premenstrual syndrome (PMS). And after a hysterectomy, women with heightened levels of depression may be said to have 'post-hysterectomy depression' syndrome. While not disputing that disturbances of reproductive function can affect mood and behaviour, and that the obverse may also apply, it must be said that many of the associations suggested to date seem oversimplified.

Doctors have suggested for many years that menopausal depression is a depressive disorder occurring specifically in the mid-life years and that it is different from other depressive disorders. Little evidence has, however, been found to support this idea. Studies have actually found high levels of well-being among women during mid-life.[10] And, as far as hysterectomised women are concerned, there is little evidence that they are any more prone to depression after hysterectomy than before. In those cases where menopausal women are diagnosed as having psychiatric symptoms, there is a stronger association with important life events, relationships with children, and marital status than with cessation of menstruation. Furthermore, some women experience physical symptoms such as hot flushes without any psychiatric symptoms, while the reverse is true for others.

There is still much to learn about these associations as many of the studies carried out to date have involved small numbers of self-selected women rather than large random samples. The Melbourne Women's Midlife Health Project is an attempt to overcome some of these deficiencies. It aims to help rectify a situation where the linkages described are, in the words of the United States Office of Technology Assessment, 'based on myths, unwarranted assumptions and conclusions derived from outdated, poorly constructed studies'.[11]

Menstrual patterns

The bleeding patterns of women as they approach menopause are as individual as women themselves. For some women, periods become lighter and less frequent until they disappear altogether. For others, periods are longer, heavier, and more frequent. This sort of bleeding, along with the pain that may accompany menstrual periods, is one of the most common reasons for women to have a hysterectomy. Factors known to affect women's bleeding patterns include their weight, race, nutritional factors, such as the fat content of their diet, and hormonal influences, which may be inherited or introduced into their lifestyle as hormones in the form of tablets, injections, implants, patches or ointments. Studies in progress are examining other theories for why unexpected bleeding patterns occur.

Sometimes women bleed after their menopause, that is, after not having had a period for more than a year. If this occurs, it is essential that it be checked by a competent medical practitioner as it may indicate the presence of a serious, perhaps even life-threatening, disorder such as cancer. In the case of Susan, spots of blood appeared on her underwear at the age of fifty-eight, six years after her menopause. Initially, she thought wear and tear during intercourse might be responsible for the spotting, but when it continued and bore no apparent relation to when she had sex, she raised the matter with her doctor. A vaginal cream containing oestrogen that Susan had been using for three years to reduce vaginal dryness was the probable culprit. However the doctor conducted vaginal and pelvic examinations and took a Pap smear before taking a specimen of cells from the endometrium (a gynoscan). This showed that the endometrium had become quite thick, which can occur when vaginal creams containing oestrogen are used after menopause. The gynaecologist performed a dilatation and curettage (D and C, see chapter 3) to remove the endometrial build-up and reduced the dosage of oestrogen in the cream she was using to ensure that the same problem did not recur.

Uterus movement

If you picture the uterus as an organ that is essentially static in the abdomen, think again. The combination of elastic tissue and muscle in the supporting ligaments of

Figure 3   Possible orientations of the uterus

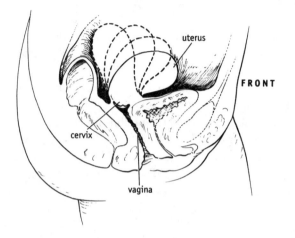

the uterus is organised to enable rapid adjustment to the altered position and size of its neighbouring organs, the bladder, bowel and vagina (figure 3). When the bladder or rectum is full, the uterus moves accordingly. In addition, the uterus lifts out of the way with the entry of the penis into the vagina during sexual intercourse. In this position, the uterus may contract during orgasm. When a woman lies on her back, the uterus hugs the rear of the pelvis; if she rolls onto her stomach, it moves towards her belly button; and when she stands, the uterus drops down a centimetre or two, a movement that is accentuated if she has a prolapse and the ligaments do not provide strong support for the uterus.

Displacement of the uterus also occurs if there is a lump or growth in a neighbouring organ. For example, a lump in the vagina pushes the uterus upwards. On the other hand, if there is a growth in the bowel the uterus is pushed forwards, and in the bladder, backwards. The uterus is also able to rotate around the point where the cervix meets the rest of the body. A forwards rotation is called anteversion, and a backwards rotation, retroversion. Some women find these movements uncomfortable if they occur during sexual activity or when a doctor is examining their uterus to see if its ability to move is restricted in any way. In most cases women are largely unaware of these movements, although they may account for some of the pelvic 'twinges' or abdominal pain that is sometimes experienced.

For the uterus to contract successfully — which occurs during menstrual bleeds, childbirth and, in perhaps a third of women, during orgasm — the muscle tissue of the uterus and of the surrounding ligaments must work harmoniously. Women do not have conscious control over these contractions; this is exercised by nerves and hormones. Some aspects of uterine function are under dual control of both hormones and nerves, while others are influenced mainly by one or the other.

two

Why women consider a hysterectomy

There are many reasons why hysterectomies are carried out, the most common being fibroids and unexplained heavy menstrual bleeding. Australian Institute of Health and Welfare studies indicate that fibroids account for about 6500 (22%) and heavy menstrual bleeding for about 5300 (18%) of the estimated 30 000 hysterectomies performed in Australia each year.[1] In the US, fibroids are said to be responsible for as many as 30% of hysterectomies and a further 20% are due to excessive bleeding of uncertain cause.[2] Other major reasons given for the hysterectomies performed in Australia are prolapse (7–21% depending on the type of hospital and State in which it is located), endometriosis and adenomyosis (6–23%), cancer (1–12%) and pelvic inflammatory disease (2–8%).[3] Multiple reasons are given for the remaining hysterectomies.

While information is available about the number of women who have hysterectomies and the underlying reasons, much greater uncertainty surrounds the women who consider the option of hysterectomy but decide against it. It is probable that these women number many, many thousands.

Uterine fibroids (myomas)

These knobs of muscle tissue grow from the lining of the uterus into its interior, from the outer surface of the uterus, or they may be buried in the myometrium, the muscular wall of the uterus (figure 4). They vary from the size of pumpkin seeds to oranges, although they can become even bigger, and usually grow slowly. They can cause excessive bleeding, pelvic pain, back pain and symptoms related to the pressure they exert on nearby organs, such as the bladder, bowel or rectum. Fibroid complications include urinary frequency (if fibroids are exerting significant pressure on the bladder), haemorrhoids or varicose veins in the legs (when the rectal or pelvic veins are squashed), and constipation (when the pressure is to the bowel).

Fibroids do not spread outside the uterus and are not a form of cancer. On very rare occasions a fibroid develops into a sarcoma, which is a cancer capable of spreading into various parts of the body. If fibroid growth is exceptionally rapid, a sarcoma may be suspected. Fibroids normally shrink after menopause. This post-menopausal decline in size is an important phenomenon because it means that 'toughing out' fibroid problems until menopause provides a solution for some women. The option of 'watchful waiting' as menopause approaches is discussed in chapter 3.

Although widely referred to as fibroids, doctors may also describe these growths as uterine fibroid tumours, uterine leiomyomas, fibroid polyps, fibromas, myomas, fibroleiomyomas or fibromyomas. It has been estimated that around 20% of women over the age of thirty have one or more fibroids in their uterus; but in many cases these do not cause problems and are never discovered. Suspicion about the presence of a fibroid or fibroids in

Figure 4 Possible sites of fibroid growth

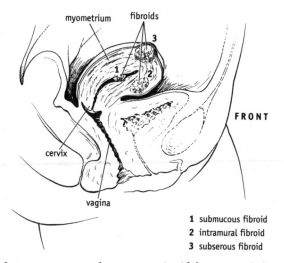

1 submucous fibroid
2 intramural fibroid
3 subserous fibroid

other women may, however, arise if the uterus is inexplicably enlarged or if menstrual periods become consistently heavier than in earlier years.

For about a third of women with fibroids the amount of blood lost during menstruation is a problem that may be accompanied by anaemia. This means there are fewer than normal red blood cells in the bloodstream, leading to a low haemoglobin level and associated fatigue, weakness and, in very severe cases, heart palpitations or heart pain (angina). Even when fibroids are small they can lead to problems of heavy bleeding, pelvic pain, back pain and urinary frequency. The reasons why fibroids sometimes cause pelvic pain are uncertain but may include the twisting of the fibroid back on itself, degenerative changes to or infection of the fibroid, or the growth of a large fibroid which the uterus tries to push out, especially during menstruation.

Lena's main problem with fibroids was painful, heavy, clot-laden bleeding which occurred for eight or more

days each month. After almost a year of putting up with this, she felt frustrated about the situation and was determined to do something about it. When a friend mentioned the possibility of a hysterectomy, she had strong reservations. She wanted to have a child, and her doctor agreed that a myomectomy (the surgical removal of fibroids from the uterus, see chapter 3) was appropriate in her case. This was carried out successfully, leaving her uterus intact. Some years later, by which time Lena had given birth to a child, the fibroids recurred. This time they were even more troublesome causing pain and severe haemorrhoids as well as heavy bleeding. An internal examination revealed that the fibroids were more extensive and intrusive than they had been previously and Lena decided on a hysterectomy (see chapter 4).

Before a diagnosis of fibroids is confirmed, other possible reasons for a mass in the abdomen should be excluded; for example, pregnancy or cancer of the cervix, endometrium or ovaries. To rule out pregnancy in a premenopausal woman, a sample of blood or urine is tested and a result obtained within minutes. To exclude cancer, several diagnostic procedures may be necessary. These include a Pap smear; a colposcopy, which entails viewing the cervix with a magnifying instrument called a colposcope, with or without removing a small sample of tissue (a biopsy) for subsequent examination; dilatation and curettage, in which the cervix is stretched or dilated and an instrument is inserted to scrape away most of the uterine lining; an ultrasound examination conducted via the vagina which produces an image of the uterus and other internal structures; and laparoscopy, a pelvic examination using a laparoscope (a tubular instrument with a light at one end and an eyepiece at the other) inserted through a small incision in the abdominal wall. Before committing to a diagnosis a doctor may also want to exclude other situations in which similar symptoms can occur, such as endometriosis, a pregnancy in a Fallopian tube, irregular placement of the uterus, bladder cancer, and ascites, which is an accumulation of fluid in the abdomen.

Doctors do not usually recommend removing fibroids if they are not causing problems, and it is estimated that this is the situation for most women who have them. In these women, fibroids tend to be diagnosed during a routine check-up, usually causing suspicion because the uterus is larger than expected but there is no evidence of pregnancy. If a doctor feels a firm, irregularly shaped mass when conducting an abdominal examination, the likelihood is that one or more fibroids are present.

When suggestions are made about removing fibroids that are not producing symptoms, this may be because of concerns that their further growth could make later removal difficult, or could result in serious complications by pressing on nearby organs. Of course doctors do not have crystal balls and predicting which patients will experience a worsening of their symptoms requires a good deal of guesswork. If this is the reason given for hysterectomy, it should be closely questioned. It is reasonable to remove symptomless fibroids if they are blocking the cervix, protruding into the uterine cavity or closing off the Fallopian tubes. Recent estimates suggest that fibroids are involved in about one in fifty cases of infertility in Australian couples.

The cause or causes of fibroids are uncertain although it is clear that stimulation of the myometrium by oestrogen promotes their growth and development. When oestrogen levels are high, as occurs during the reproductive years in general and pregnancy in particular, fibroids tend to increase in size. When oestrogen levels fall, for example after menopause, fibroids tend to shrink. During the past decade, further valuable insights have emerged. Studies of large population groups show that fibroids are much more common in women from certain racial groups. Black women in the US, for example, are three to nine times more likely to develop fibroids than comparable White women. Suspicion has fallen on genetic factors and pelvic infections, but it has also been suggested that a predisposition to fibroid formation occurs in obese women with above-average levels of blood glucose and growth hormone. Oestrogen and growth hormone are synergistic, meaning that their combined effect is greater than the effect of either hormone acting alone. Women on the Pill and those who smoke cigarettes seem to be less likely to develop fibroids.

A variety of approaches to managing fibroids and associated bleeding problems, without resorting to hysterectomy, are described in the next chapter. These include 'watchful waiting' for fibroids, drug therapies, hysteroscopic resection, myomectomy, herbal therapies and cauterisation.

Heavy, prolonged menstrual periods

As many as 10% of healthy women experience menstrual bleeding during their lives that seems heavier, more prolonged and perhaps also more painful than anything they can remember from previous years. Women describe the experience in many ways: 'I'm flooding at least once a day', 'I'm passing clots', 'My periods go on and on', 'They're much heavier and more painful than they used to be'.

Women with no previous gynaecological problems, and no reason to think they have fibroids, polyps, a pelvic infection or endometriosis, are in a quandary. Are these bleeding episodes a cause for concern? Or are they a normal response to changing levels of sex hormones, perhaps associated with menopause-related changes, or to something else? Most women experience irregular menstrual periods for between two and seven years prior to menopause, although the range is a few months to eleven years. This can be a stressful time because of concerns about the cause of the bleeding.

Doctors classify excessive heavy bleeding (menorrhagia) as the repeated loss of more than 80 ml of menstrual blood in each menstrual cycle. If this volume is lost consistently during menstruation, women can become anaemic, lethargic and prone to sickness. While this is a concern for health reasons, the social impact is often more worrying still, with the added burden of possibly creating financial difficulties. Some women find they need to plan their activities carefully to minimise the embarrassment of bleeding accidents, or they may take time off work coping with the problem or trying to find out the underlying cause. **Kath's experience of heavy bleeding coincided with a very hot summer. After a couple of bleeding accidents when she 'flooded' on her way to, or at, work she took the precaution of wearing dark-coloured clothing that would disguise any such episode, as well as using tampons and sanitary pads of increased absorbency. A number of colleagues unwittingly added to her embarrassment by making disparaging comments about the inappropriateness of her clothing given the sweltering heat. Initially Kath tried to shrug the comments off and joked about getting dressed** before the lights came on. But one day she decided enough was enough and, when quizzed about her clothing, she simply said, 'I'm having a hellish time with my periods at the moment and, believe me, I'll be celebrating when I can wear white again.'

Difficulties with heavy bleeding can be compounded by serious problems on the home-front, as exemplified by Sara Henderson, the irrepressible co-owner of a cattle station in outback Australia. Sara recalls in her autobiography, *From Strength to Strength*, that at the age of fifty, and at a time of great personal and financial stress, her periods threatened to land her in hospital. They were up to ten days long and had become noticeably heavier at around the time she was nursing her estranged husband after major surgery and visiting her elderly mother who had become partially paralysed following a stroke. Fortunately Sara's worst bleeding episode was swiftly stemmed by a single injection (see chapter 3).

In normal day to day living, measuring how much blood is lost in a menstrual bleed is virtually impossible. When careful studies are conducted, however, women are found to lose about 35 ml of blood (less than a quarter of a cup) in a cycle on average. Clearly, the 80 ml marker of menorrhagia is set quite high.

The diagnosis of excessive heavy bleeding is usually based on a joint assessment by women and their doctors. Factors taken into account include the number and degree of saturation of pads and/or tampons, the duration of bleeding, and the presence or absence of clots and flooding. This assessment is subjective and various research studies suggest that women may think they are losing more or less blood than is revealed by a careful analysis of sanitary products. In one study, for example, while 59% of women with concerns about menorrhagia were losing more than 60 ml of blood in most cycles, another 20% had average losses of less than 35 ml.[4] Younger women in particular seem to be more likely to regard moderate blood loss as heavy. Reassurance about bleeding patterns, if this is appropriate, or information about how to better organise and cope with tampon and pad use (see chapter 3) can result in management of the problem without drugs or surgery.

A specific cause for heavy bleeding may never be found, although there is usually much speculation about possible reasons. Fibroids are thought to be the culprit in about a quarter of cases, while in others polyps, endometriosis, polycystic ovaries, abnormalities of the body's blood-clotting mechanism, chronic liver or kidney disease, ectopic pregnancy, pelvic inflammatory disease, and side-effects from hormone therapies and intra-uterine contraceptive devices are implicated. Where possible, likely causes should be avoided, removed or treated.

Where there is no explanation for recurrent heavy blood loss, doctors usually describe the bleeding as 'dysfunctional'. Drug therapies or removal (resection) of the endometrium (both dealt with in chapter 3) are the usual strategies in trying to correct the problem. If these approaches do not work, a hysterectomy may be the last resort.

Prolapse

Weaknesses in the vagina and in the ligaments supporting the bladder, rectum and uterus can cause the 'dropping' of a pelvic organ, which is known as a prolapse (figure 5). The symptoms depend on the type of prolapse but commonly there is a sensation of something coming down the vagina or a lump within it, or low back pain which improves on lying flat. Pain during sexual inter-

Figure 5   Cross-section of the body showing first-degree uterine prolapse. Refer to figure 2(a) for a comparison with the uterus in normal position

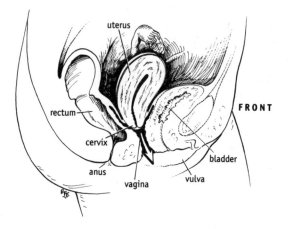

course (dyspareunia, pronounced dis-puh-roon-ea) may also occur.

The main reasons for prolapse are difficult childbirth, other types of damage to the pelvic support structures (sometimes brought about by a hysterectomy itself), ageing processes in tissues and inherited defects of the pelvic support tissues. Women who have a chronic cough or constipation seem particularly vulnerable to prolapse.

When a doctor refers to a 'uterine prolapse' this means that a weakness in the uterine support structures has caused the uterus to drop into the vagina, causing that tissue to move downwards. A 'first degree uterine prolapse' means the cervix is 'low', being within easy reach of a finger inserted in the vagina. In second degree prolapse, the cervix has dropped to be near the vaginal entrance. Occasionally, the uterus is completely prolapsed, which means the cervix appears at the vaginal entrance. This third degree prolapse condition is known as procidentia (pronounced pro-see-dench-ea) or uterine descent. Sitting and walking are understandably difficult and, if the protruding cervix chafes during walking, this can cause a blood-stained discharge.

Other sorts of prolapse are often described under the umbrella-term, 'vaginal prolapse'. They are described as:

- cystocele, in which part of the bladder drops into the vagina
- enterocele, when a loop of intestine does the same thing
- urethrocele, where the urethra (the 3–4 cm long canal through which urine passes from the bladder to the urethral opening near the entrance to the vagina) presses into the vagina
- cystourethrocele, where a cystocele and a urethrocele occur together
- rectocele, in which the wall of the rectum protrudes into the vagina.

In the case of a cystocele, urethrocele or cystourethrocele, bladder weakness is common as well as the general feeling of downward pressure in the vagina (women often liken the feeling to a lump coming down or out of the vagina). Leakage of urine may occur on coughing, laughing or sneezing, and urinary tract infections may be a recurring problem. A rectocele can produce a feeling of incomplete emptying of the rectum as a pocket of tissue may form which traps faecal matter. Some women find they can complete their bowel action by pressing firmly on the bridge of tissue between the vaginal opening and the anus.

The incident which prompted 37-year-old Marjorie to visit her doctor was an evening out with friends during which she had laughed long and loud. She felt the leakage of a small amount of urine and became

embarrassed and uncomfortable. Visualising a patch on her dress that her friends and partner would see if she stood up, she spent twenty agonising minutes glued to the chair until an opportunity to casually leave the room arose. Her local doctor asked Marjorie to complete a urinary diary for a week and diagnosed a cysto- cele after a full pelvic examination, including a rectal examination.

Prolapse carries no risk to life, provided there is no urinary tract obstruction or current infection of the urinary tract. If prolapse is not causing symptoms, watching and waiting to check on progression is a reas- onable approach. Medical as well as surgical treatments are available if necessary, and choosing the best approach depends on factors like a woman's age, state of health, and her desire to have children and to retain the ability to have sex. If surgery is not suitable, a supporting plastic or rubber device called a pessary can be inserted in the va- gina to support the uterus in its normal position. Women with uterine prolapse or a cystocele may be helped by ring pessaries, made of inert plastic. These can remain in place for several months without removal and cleaning, provided they do not produce any adverse effects such as a smelly vaginal discharge. Considerable improvement may be achieved when the pessary is combined with a vaginal oestrogen ointment and exercises to strengthen the pelvic floor.

Surgery for prolapse problems dates back more than a century and recent advances include techniques to repair muscles and ligaments, and repositioning of the pelvic organs. In some cases a vaginal hysterectomy (see chap- ter 4) may be suggested. The choice of surgical approach may be affected if a woman wants to remain sexually active, so this should be discussed with her doctor at an early stage.

Chronic pelvic pain and period pain

Chronic pelvic pain is associated with as many as 10% of hysterectomies but its cause is uncertain.[5] Some studies suggest that there may be a link between this type of pain and psychological factors or a history of childhood sexual abuse. Investigation of the underlying cause usually entails a pelvic examination, laparoscopy, and ultrasound or magnetic resonance imaging (MRI) investigations. These can help rule out the presence of fibroids, endometriosis, adenomyosis, disorders of the ovaries and Fallopian tubes, and pelvic inflammatory disease. When no cause is identified for the pain, medical treatments such as nonsteroidal anti-inflammatory agents and the contraceptive Pill (see chapter 3) are often tried, with hysterectomy (chapter 4) being the last resort when pain is so severe that it is disrupting everyday activities and seriously diminishing quality of life.

There are two main types of period pain or dysmenorrhoea (pronounced dis-men-or-eea). Primary dysmenorrhoea usually affects young women who have never been pregnant. It begins when bleeding starts or just beforehand and rarely lasts more than twenty-four hours. The pain is cramp-like and is usually felt in the lower abdomen, lower back or the insides of the thighs. Occasionally it is so severe that it causes fainting, nausea or vomiting. The cause of the pain is linked to an increase in contraction of the uterus. This may be related to excessive secretions of prostaglandin substances by the endometrium or an increased sensitivity of the uterus to them, causing stronger contractions. Secondary dysmenorrhoea is more often experienced by women whose periods have been painless for some years. The pain may last throughout the menstrual bleeding phase and is thought to be a symptom of something amiss in the reproductive system, for example tissue inflammation, endometriosis, pelvic infection or fibroids. Drugs with anti-prostaglandin activity are often used to treat dysmenorrhoea (see chapter 3); in severe cases of primary dysmenorrhoea the pain can be stopped by the inhibition of ovulation through hormone treatments such as the contraceptive Pill.

Endometriosis

Endometriosis is the growth of tissue resembling the endometrium in parts of the pelvis where it is not usually seen (figure 6). This 'stray' tissue grows in an estimated 1–6% of women. It occurs on the ovaries, Fallopian tubes, the outside of the uterus or its supporting liga-

Figure 6   Growth of endometriosis tissue on the reproductive organs

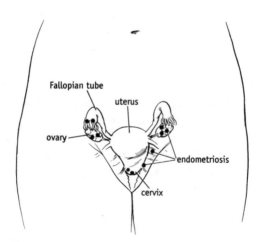

ments, the bowel, bladder or vagina.[6] It occurs in about one in five women with fertility problems, suggesting a significant role in infertility. The tissue behaves like the endometrium in some respects, bleeding at the same time as the usual menstrual period. If the blood cannot easily escape from the body, it may cause irritation or pain and may develop into blood-filled cysts.

Sometimes endometriosis only lasts for a few cycles, but it may also continue throughout reproductive life, getting worse as women enter their thirties and forties. The behaviour of endometriosis in pregnancy is highly variable and it rarely disappears permanently after pregnancy. Published reports indicate that some women continue to have problems due to endometriosis after menopause. It can limit bending, stretching, standing and taking exercise, especially on days of menstrual bleeding. Although it is also associated with infertility, many women with endometriosis become pregnant without difficulty.

Endometriosis is regarded as the most common cause of chronic pain in women aged from fifteen to fifty-five years. This pain is nearly always cyclical, that is, it tends to occur at about the same time in most menstrual cycles. It may be experienced by a woman when she ovulates, menstruates or is about to menstruate. It may also occur when she has sexual intercourse, urinates or passes a bowel motion. It sometimes causes spotting between periods. Although it has much in common with period pain it does not respond to medications, such as anti-prostaglandins, found helpful in that disorder. **When Laura sought advice from her doctor about chronic pelvic pain, a number of factors in her history suggested a diagnosis of endometriosis. These included a history of painful periods which had worsened with age, short menstrual cycles with a relatively large number of days** of bleeding, and a family history of pelvic pain among her female relatives. Despite this suggestive evidence, Laura's doctor advised her that the diagnosis required a laparoscopy, entailing a visual inspection of her abdominal organs. He said a number of other procedures might assist in arriving at a diagnosis but he preferred not to perform a biopsy of suspected lesions, a vaginal ultrasound and blood tests until he did the laparoscopy. In fact, the laparoscopy was sufficient to reveal the endometriosis and he and Laura discussed a number of possible treatments, including drug treatment and surgical removal (see chapter 3).

The diagnosis of endometriosis usually relies on a laparoscopic examination, a procedure that enables a doctor to examine the contents of the abdomen without making a big opening in it (see figure 13). Instead several small incisions are made and a long thin tube specially equipped with thin glass fibres is inserted through one of the incisions. Light travels along the fibres to 'spotlight' internal organs and a periscope-type attachment allows the doctor to see into the abdomen and pelvis. Other instruments used with the laparoscope (hence the need for the other incisions) enable the doctor to make photographic records of the inside of the abdomen, obtain samples (biopsies) of tissue for laboratory analysis and remove abnormal tissue. Using this technique, doctors have learned that the appearance of endometriosis varies markedly. Younger women tend to have clear growths or red lesions, whereas the lesions of older patients tend to be black or yellow-white.

Various theories have been advanced about why endometriosis occurs, but these are hotly disputed. Suffice it to say that no one yet knows if some women are born with a tendency to develop it or if endometrial-type tissue spreads in the body due to some unusual abdominal structure or function. Treatments for endometriosis, including drug therapies and surgery, are described in chapter 3.

Adenomyosis

Adenomyosis refers to endometriosis growing within the thick muscular coat of the uterus, the myometrium. The symptoms include enlargement of the uterus, and heavy or painful bleeding, and the group of women affected is similar to that for endometriosis. Its presence may be suggested by vaginal ultrasound, biopsy of the myometrium or magnetic resonance imaging .

While it is sometimes possible to remove endometriosis by cutting or burning it out (see chapter 3), this is more difficult where adenomyosis is concerned. Drug therapies (also discussed in chapter 3) can provide profound pain relief for both endometriosis and adenomyosis while in use, but there is no evidence that they eradicate the unwanted tissue. After therapy stops, the disease persists in more than three out of four women and pain often recurs within a few weeks or months. Many women consider hysterectomy (chapter 4) when endometriosis or adenomyosis continues to cause severe and persistent problems despite other treatments.

Cancer

Cancer of the cervix

There are several sites for cancer that prompt women to consider a hysterectomy. Cancer of the cervix, also called cervical cancer, develops in cells that line the cervix. The abnormal changes usually occur over a period of years, although in some women the changes seem to happen much faster. Abnormalities of the cells of the cervix, thought to be precursors of cervical cancer, used to be called dysplasia; but nowadays the term cervical intra-epithelial neoplasia (CIN) is used.

Cervical cancer is diagnosed in about 1100 Australian women each year. Although most diagnoses are made in women aged over fifty-five, it seems that increasing numbers of women in their twenties and thirties are now being affected. Tell-tale signs include bleeding between periods in pre-menopausal women, bleeding after sexual intercourse or at any time after menopause, and a smelly vaginal discharge.

Screening for cervical cell abnormalities that could develop into cancer is available using the Pap smear technique. A small sample or biopsy of cells from the cervix is obtained using a special brush and a fine wooden spatula. The cells are smeared onto a piece of glass and then sent to a laboratory for examination. From the appearance of the cells, it is possible to identify cancer at a stage early enough to permit its complete removal and cure. Australian health authorities recommend a Pap smear every second year from the time women start to be sexually active.

Over 400 000 women in the State of Victoria, Australia, had a Pap smear during 1990, but seven out of ten women considered to be most at risk of cervical cancer did not come forward for testing. Of every ten smears done, eight were completely normal or showed insignificant changes. Less than four in every 100 smears showed CIN changes and only one in every 2000 was suggestive of possible cancer. If the results of a Pap smear raise concerns, or if a woman experiences any unusual bleeding or cervical discharge, the cervix is examined for suspicious-looking tissue using a magnifying instrument called a colposcope. A biopsy is usually taken and the tissue sample removed from the cervix is sent to a laboratory for microscopic examination. If the examination indicates severe CIN or pre-invasive cancer, any areas of the cervix which look abnormal are treated by cryosurgery (which destroys tissue by freezing), diathermy (which achieves the same end using an electric current), or else by heat or by laser. Diathermy or electrocoagulation entails using an electric current to produce points, loops or small balls of heat that burn the tissue while also closing blood vessels. Lasers are high-density beams of light energy that can cut tissue precisely and, at the same time, close off blood vessels. All these techniques have a high cure rate, and they do not interfere with a woman's sex life or prevent her from having children in the future. Occasionally, a procedure called conisation is performed in which a cone-shaped sample of tissue about a centimetre thick is removed from the cervix using a scalpel, diathermy or laser. Once again, it is rare for the technique to damage a woman's sex life or impair her ability to have children. If, however, there is any evidence that the disease has spread inside or beyond the cervix, a hysterectomy (see chapter 4) should be discussed. Radiation therapy or chemotherapy may also be suggested in a bid to ensure the complete destruction of cancer cells.

Although scientists do not know the exact cause of cervical cancer, there appears to be an association with sexual activity. Research suggests that certain strains of the human papilloma virus (HPV), which may be transferred during sexual contact, are involved in the disease process.

Cancer of the endometrium

This form of cancer arises in the lining of the uterus and is diagnosed in approximately 1000 Australian women each year. Most are aged between fifty and sixty-five, and those affected are more likely than average to have diabetes or high blood pressure, to be overweight, to have polycystic ovarian syndrome or to have continued menstruating beyond the age of fifty. Women who have never had children and those who are on oestrogen after menopause without also using a progestogen are also at higher risk. This is why many doctors are reluctant to prescribe oestrogen on its own in pill, patch or implant form to women with a uterus, preferring to add progestogen hormone to protect the endometrium. (They may, however, safely prescribe forms of oestrogen that are made for absorption through the vagina such as creams and pessaries, as long as these are limited to two or three applications a week.)

As only about half the women who develop endometrial cancer are in identified high risk groups, it is vital that all women are aware of tell-tale symptoms of the disease. The most common sign of endometrial cancer is unusual bleeding. This means any sort of bleeding — including just a few spots of blood — for women who have gone through menopause. For women who are still menstruating, it means unusually heavy bleeding during, or between, periods.

Diagnosis usually involves one of two techniques, aspiration curettage or D and C. Aspiration curettage is a simple procedure that can be performed in a doctor's office. A thin tube is inserted through the cervix into the uterus and a small sample of endometrial tissue is obtained under suction. This can then be sent to a laboratory for examination. If a D and C is performed, a general anaesthetic is usually required. The cervix is stretched, or dilated, and a small instrument inserted into the uterus. Cells from the endometrium are scraped off and this sample is sent for laboratory examination.

If early pre-cancerous changes are detected, the situation is usually watched carefully to make sure that they do not develop. More serious pre-cancerous changes may warrant an endometrial resection (see chapter 3) or the triggering of a period using a medical therapy (also described in chapter 3). A woman with a uterus who is using oestrogen on its own either needs to add progesterone to her hormone intake (for at least part of the cycle) or she should be prepared to have endometrial biopsies on a regular basis.

If cancerous changes are evident in the endometrium an abdominal or vaginal hysterectomy is usually performed, with or without radiotherapy, chemotherapy and progestogen hormone therapy. Endometrial cancer detected in its early stages can be treated successfully about 75% of the time. The outlook is poor if the cancer has spread beyond the uterus.

Cancer of the ovary

Although cancer of the ovary is less common than cancer of the cervix or endometrium, it is by no means rare. About 900 women in Australia receive this unwelcome diagnosis each year, with most of those affected aged in their sixties, seventies and eighties. On average, about one Australian woman in every 100 will develop ovarian cancer during her lifetime. It is more common in women with infertility problems and also in some families, and less common in women on the contraceptive pill. Because few if any symptoms may be apparent early on, the cancer is usually at an advanced stage when it is diagnosed. At present only 15–25% of diagnoses are made when the cancer is limited to the ovaries. The result is that ovarian cancer is among the most lethal of the cancers affecting women. Less than a third of women survive five years from diagnosis.

Until recently, an early diagnosis — with the cancer localised in the ovaries — was usually the result of an examination for an unrelated problem. New blood tests are, however, being developed that are capable of detecting evidence of some types of ovarian cancer. Advances in ultrasound imaging techniques also offer hope that an early warning system for ovarian cancer will become available in the near future.

The cause of ovarian cancer is uncertain, but studies indicate that women with a close relative who has had the cancer (a sister, mother or daughter) and those with a history of fertility problems are at increased risk of developing it. Pill users seem to be at lower than average risk. The surgical removal of both ovaries (oophorectomy) is usual even if only one ovary seems to be diseased. A hysterectomy may be suggested because of the proximity of the uterus to the ovaries. However the desirability of a hysterectomy has to be weighed up for each woman. Chemotherapy or radiation therapy, and sometimes both, may be helpful.

Cancers of the colon, rectum and bladder

Women having surgery to remove cancers of the colon, rectum or bladder may be advised that removing the uterus will improve their prospects of survival. Unless there is evidence that the cancer has spread to the uterus and ovaries, this seems like an unnecessarily aggressive approach. Any decision to have a hysterectomy in these circumstances should take account of the long-term impacts of hysterectomy on an individual woman's physical and emotional well-being.

Pelvic inflammatory disease or infection

Inflammation of women's reproductive organs is referred to as pelvic inflammatory disease (PID). When the

Fallopian tubes are affected, the condition is called salpingitis. Pus produced in the tubes or other organs in response to the inflammation may interfere with their normal function and result in symptoms of abdominal pain, fever and tenderness. Any one of a number of micro-organisms may be responsible for PID and it is thought that these are sexually transmitted. PID tends to occur in women who have had many sexual partners or women whose partners have had many sexual partners.

Prompt treatment of PID with antibiotics can bring rapid relief from discomfort. Recurrent episodes of PID can, however, result in irreversible damage to the Fallopian tubes (causing problems with fertility) and persistent symptoms. Techniques to clear blocked Fallopian tubes and restore them to good health are sometimes successful in restoring fertility and reducing pain. These techniques include hysteroscopic tubal cannulation, falloposcopy and microsurgery. If severe PID is resistant to treatment and the woman concerned has no desire to become pregnant in the future, removal of the uterus, ovaries and Fallopian tubes may be considered (see chapter 4).

Pelvic adhesions

Infections and surgical procedures are common causes of adhesions, which are filmy or thick strands of scar tissue that bind organs together. Adhesions can develop between the uterus, ovaries, bowel, bladder and rectum because of their proximity in the abdomen. Pain can occur any time that adhesions are stretched, for example during movement, a pelvic examination, sexual intercourse, passing urine or a bowel motion. If adhesions are constricting the ovary, pain may occur only, or mainly, during ovulation; if constricting the bladder, the pain may be intense when the bladder is full, easing as the bladder empties. Adhesions can also result in infertility by constricting the Fallopian tubes, covering or displacing the ovaries, or impeding the movement of sperm and egg or interfering with the growth of embryos. Ironically, while hysterectomy is sometimes successful in overcoming pain caused by adhesions, hysterectomy itself may be responsible for severe adhesions that result in long-term pain and intestinal obstruction.

The diagnosis of pelvic adhesions in a woman relies mainly on her history of infections or surgery and the nature of her pain. The diagnosis is usually confirmed by laparoscopy, although ultrasound can be useful in revealing adhesions surrounding the ovaries or bowel. If laparoscopy is performed in the presence of extensive adhesions it can result in puncture of the bowel, so great care must be taken with this technique and alternative methods (such as a mini-laparotomy) may have to be considered. (A mini-laparotomy entails a small incision through the abdominal wall to allow inspection of the internal organs. It is like a mini-Caesarean section.)

It is possible to remove adhesions without going to the lengths of hysterectomy in most women, and one of the most useful techniques is laparoscopic surgery. The laparoscope or viewing tube (for inspecting the internal organs) is used in conjunction with fine forceps which can hold the adhesions steady or break them with a blunt action, scissors to cut the adhesions, lasers to vaporise them, or high frequency electrical currents that produce heat and destroy them. In order to minimise adhesion formation, it is important that your surgeon is gentle and careful in his or her handling of the tissues, that techniques are used to prevent bleeding, and that solutions or special membranes to reduce adhesion formation and other complications are used in the abdomen.

Post-pregnancy complications

Emergency hysterectomy may be the only option when uterine bleeding is uncontrollable. This is a rare occurrence after childbirth and may be caused by rupture of the uterus or damage to major blood vessels. Other situations that may give rise to hysterectomy include life-threatening infection of the endometrium (a very occasional complication of abortion), or the removal of an ectopic pregnancy in a woman who has finished her family.

Severe premenstrual syndrome

Many women in their fertile years become moody and tense and feel 'down' in the week before their menstrual periods. In about 2–8% of women these changes are severe. They may also feel hopeless and angry, may be easily distracted and disinterested in work, friends and hobbies. In addition, their breasts may feel swollen, their heads may ache, their abdomens may feel bloated, and their joints and muscles painful. Difficulties with sleepiness or sleeplessness may also pose problems. Within a few days of starting to menstruate, these difficulties diminish or disappear.

Women for whom these sorts of changes occur at a predictable time in most menstrual cycles may be suffering from premenstrual syndrome. Hormonal changes during the menstrual cycle are sometimes blamed for the condition but it seems there is also a strong psychological component. Distress from other sources, such as marriage, parenthood or occupation, may interact with hormonal changes resulting in intermittent negative moods and behaviours.

Patricia, a 35-year-old mother, sought help for severe irritability, uncontrolled anger, confusion, insomnia, fatigue and low libido, which typically appeared two weeks before her period and disappeared about a week after bleeding stopped. With a thirty day menstrual cycle, this meant she experienced only about eight days when she felt well and 'in control' of her situation. Doctors occasionally suggest a hysterectomy in such circum-stances in a bid to relieve symptoms that are disrupting relationships and generally making life a misery. There is, however, little evidence to support the value of this approach as symptoms often persist after hysterectomy.

Patricia found a coping skills program incorporating anxiety-reduction techniques and responsible assertive-ness training to be extremely helpful. Within twelve weeks she was increasingly positive about her relation-ships in all directions and regarded her premenstrual phase as a time when she felt 'out of sorts' but from which she would recover her competence within a day or two.

Permanent contraception and relief from bleeding

Women who have difficulty with contraception or who, for religious reasons, do not want to use drugs or devices to control their fertility sometimes find themselves in a situation of despair regarding family planning. They may have as many children as they can cope with and may feel that a hysterectomy is the only way out of their dilemma.

Equally, hysterectomy is sometimes seen as a 'solution' to contraception worries and bleeding difficulties for disabled teenage women. **When Jane was seventeen, her case went before the Family Court. She was profoundly intellectually disabled and had epilepsy and was unable to communicate with her carers except to smile when happy and to resist when unwilling to do what they asked. Her parents had applied to the Family Court for an order allowing them to consent to a hysterectomy on her behalf. Following a 1992 decision, courts have to give permission in Australia before a non-therapeutic hysterectomy is carried out on an intellectually disabled female. They argued that it would assist in her hygiene, control her epilepsy (which worsened when she menstruated), and could prevent her becoming pregnant. The judge held that it was not in Jane's best interests to have the operation, although three of the four doctors who gave evidence disagreed.** There are no easy answers to dilemmas such as these, for the issues extend well beyond the medical into social areas.

Psychological factors

For reasons that are unclear, women who are scheduled for hysterectomy are more than twice as likely as average to be distressed as indicated by psychological tests.[7] It may be that symptoms such as chronic pain and heavy bleeding, and uncertainty about the future, have produced this psychological distress. Or else, an underlying psychological condition may have reduced tolerance of minor symptoms. Whatever the truth of the matter, improvement in gynaecological complaints, however this is achieved, tends to result in a marked reduction in psychological symptoms. On rare occasions such women may ask about, or be advised to have, a hysterectomy.

three

Alternatives to hysterectomy

Each of us responds in our own way to the experience of illness and we all have views about the sorts of treatments we find acceptable. For each there are different circumstances and different priorities. For example, women of all ages would prefer not to have bleeding accidents and may be prepared to undergo extensive investigation and difficult treatments to achieve this end. Other factors that may influence attitudes to treatment include the dollar cost, the risk of adverse effects and complications, the time to recovery, possible effects on body- and self-image and sexuality, and the presence or absence of a family history of gynaecological disease of one sort or another. Weighing up these sorts of considerations, along with input from health advisers, family, friends and other information sources, will influence our views on treatment. The challenge is to find the treatment that is most suitable and has the best outcome given particular individual situations and needs.

'Watchful waiting'

For some women, coping with difficult menstrual bleeding or painful periods without drugs or surgery is an option worthy of serious consideration. The rationale for a 'watchful waiting' approach hinges on the well-established finding that oestrogen plays a major role in the growth of fibroids and endometriosis. When oestrogen output by the ovaries decreases after menopause, these conditions tend to become much less worrying. Many women are therefore prepared to give the watchful waiting approach a try if their period problems are bearable and they are nearing menopause.

Julia experienced intermittent, heavy and painful bleeding due to fibroids for two-and-a- half years before her menopause and considered having either a myomectomy or a hysterectomy during this difficult time. Looking back some years later Julia was pleased that neither procedure was ultimately necessary. 'There were days when I felt very low because my periods were painful and flooding was an occasional embarrassment. I talked to doctors a couple of times about surgery but I mainly focused on getting through each day. I suppose I kept postponing any decision until, at last, my periods ended.'

There are many reasons for difficult-to-manage bleeding patterns apart from fibroids. Lauren had lengthy menstrual bleeds in her late forties that were different from anything she had experienced previously. During them, spotting was typical on the first few days, then there were several days of heavy bleeding which resembled the heaviest bleed of former periods, followed by a handful of days when the bleeding tapered off. Managing the blood loss was tiresome because it went on for so long and Lauren was also concerned about the possibility that something was seriously amiss. Medical investigations including a hysteroscopy (see later this chapter) did not reveal any suspicious lumps or growths and showed that she was not anaemic. Doctors said changes in her sex hormone levels, consistent with an impending menopause, were to blame for her symptoms. In order to sort out whether Lauren's blood loss was excessive, it was suggested she record what her bleeding was like. 'Keep a diary of how many days it lasts, how many and what sort of sanitary pad or tampon you use, whether pain occurs and when,' her doctor said. 'Then we'll discuss the findings.'

Lauren's diary confirmed that her blood loss was heavy and prolonged and a number of possible medical therapies were discussed as well as the option of watching and waiting. After talking with friends who had negotiated similarly difficult bleeding, Lauren decided to try a non-medical approach for a few more months. In particular, she started experimenting with dietary changes, including some herbal products (see later this chapter), and the use of highly absorbent 'overnight' sanitary pads when the bleeding was heaviest. Her boss, who had herself been through similar difficulties some years earlier, was supportive and understanding. Lauren bled profusely at night on several occasions and found it reassuring to have a mattress protector in place as well as a towel beside her bed in case of flooding. After several months her periods dwindled then stopped. 'I remember telling a doctor with pride about the range of strategies I'd used and the dismay I felt when he seemed to dismiss my efforts and talked instead of how easily my problems could have been solved with some sort of hormone therapy. He was a little more supportive when I explained that my previous experiences with the Pill were unsatisfactory, and that I wanted to avoid drug therapies if possible.'

An increasingly common cause of bleeding in the post-menopausal age group is hormone therapy. Sometimes there is no apparent reason why such problems affect one woman and not another. Occasionally the explanation seems to be pre-existing fibroids or the use of an oestrogen implant as part of post-menopausal hormone therapy. It has been noted that implants cause severe uncontrollable bleeding in some women, presumably because they deliver larger amounts of oestrogen than other hormone therapy formulations, for some of the time at least.

Another possible cause of bleeding is cancer of the endometrium in post-menopausal women who have used oestrogen therapy (in pill, patch or implant form) without added progestogen for several years. Even after oestrogen is no longer taken, the risk of cancer of the endometrium persists. It is important to seek medical advice promptly if this possibility applies to you.

Women in whom post-menopausal hormone therapy causes heavy bleeding should consult a doctor immediately as it may be prudent to reduce the dose of hormones, or switch to another form of hormone therapy (such as a patch or vaginal cream). It is important that women keep in close contact with their doctor when taking any hormone therapy. **Theresa started to bleed unpredictably and at times heavily soon after starting on an oestrogen implant and progestogen tablets. Her doctor had recommended implant therapy because of the severity of her hot flushes and vaginal dryness and because a previous stint on oestrogen tablets had caused troublesome nausea. When there was little improvement in Theresa's bleeding after four months, removal of the implant was organised and a watchful waiting approach instituted until things settled down. The doctor later prescribed oestrogen cream which Theresa applied to her vagina two or three times a week. She no longer had bleeding episodes and her vaginal lubrica-**

tion improved; although her hot flushes returned and persisted for nearly a year until they waned then disappeared.

The decision about whether to watch and wait or to try medical treatments or surgery depends on many factors including the amount of bleeding and its effect on daily living, the ability to cope with such difficulties, general health, the rate of change in conditions like fibroids, and the probable time to menopause. Situations in which watchful waiting is generally considered to be inappropriate include rapid fibroid growth resulting in a significant and measurable increase in the size of the uterus during a six-month period, bowel or urinary obstruction, and symptoms which make life seem hardly worth living.

Drug treatments for excessive bleeding

Numerous pharmaceutical treatments have been developed to stop excessive bleeding. Not only do they avoid major surgery which, until quite recently, was the only treatment option for these conditions, they also preserve a woman's fertility, a factor of increasing importance with current trends to deferral of childbearing until after the age of thirty.

In general, these treatments are best used in the short-term (that is, for no more than a year) because prolonged use tends to result in side-effects. This drug-induced respite from heavy bleeding secures time during which women and their doctors can examine the situation carefully before settling on a strategy. For women approaching menopause, medical treatments may provide just the sort of stopgap needed until their bleeding problems disappear spontaneously.

Drug treatments can shrink tissues that may be responsible for bleeding. According to some doctors this makes subsequent surgery easier; although practitioners whose approach is to cut out or excise the aberrant tissue say it makes the surgical removal of unwanted tissue more difficult because it is less visible in its shrunken form.

The cost of drug approaches compared with surgery depends on the duration of their use, whether their price is subsidised through a national health scheme (such as through the Pharmaceutical Benefits Scheme in Australia) and whether there is a need for regular medical checks or examinations.

Progestogens

Manufactured forms of the hormone progesterone, collectively known as progestogens, have been used widely to reduce menstrual blood loss. They seem to be effective in tablet form when used by women who never or rarely ovulate, who have irregular periods or confirmed endometriosis. Women prescribed progestogens should be aware that this drug is viewed negatively by some past-users because it causes fluid retention and associated nausea, weight gain, bloating, headache, mood changes and loss of libido. Any women on progestogen who has epilepsy, migraine, asthma, a heart or kidney disorder, or a history of depressive illness should have regular medical check-ups.

Combined contraceptive pill

The combined contraceptive pill (that is, all varieties that contain an oestrogen and a progestogen) has been found to reduce blood loss during menstruation in many women, including as many as three-quarters of women experiencing excessive bleeding.[1] The Pill generally reduces blood loss by about a third in women with heavy periods. It is important to note that this is not a safe option for women over thirty-five years who smoke cigarettes, as the combination of smoking plus the Pill significantly increases the risk of premature death from stroke or heart attack. Use of the Pill also increases the risk of dangerous blood clot formation (thrombosis) throughout the body, which is why women should come off the Pill a month before surgery, in the meantime using an alternative form of contraception that does not contain hormones.

Natalie went onto the Pill at the age of forty-six to 'buy time'. Her periods became heavy and painful just when her work responsibilities increased and she was under a lot of stress at home. The Pill provided Natalie with relief from menstrual distress for six months by which time her business and family crises had settled to manageable levels. She then came off the Pill and found that she could cope with her periods.

Nonsteroidal anti-inflammatory drugs

Several nonsteroidal anti-inflammatory drugs (often shortened to NSAIDs) have been used successfully to reduce excessive menstrual bleeding. The NSAIDs concerned include ibuprofen, mefenamic acid, naproxen and flurbiprofen. (Some of these substances, for example mefenamic acid, are also anti-prostaglandin drugs or prostaglandin inhibitors.) While helpful, NSAIDs are not drugs to be taken lightly. The lowest possible dose of the least toxic NSAID should be used initially as this group of drugs produces side-effects in about a third of women, resulting in nausea, vomiting, diarrhoea, headache, dizziness and rashes.

Blood clotting mechanisms

Success in halving blood loss has been reported with several drugs that act on the body's blood clotting mechanisms. They are of particular value to women with blood clotting defects. The drugs include tranexamic acid and ethamsylate. Once again, however, about a third of women on them experience side-effects of nausea, headache, dizziness, vomiting and rashes. Research studies have also raised the concern that these drugs may precipitate strokes in some women.

Danazol

This drug is also used as a treatment for endometriosis, and has been found to halve menstrual blood loss. It is often used before hysteroscopic myomectomy (see later this chapter) in order to reduce the thickness of the endometrium. The dose required to reduce bleeding (200 to 400 mg each day for three months) is less than that needed to treat endometriosis, but its side-effects can be worrying. Those of most concern include headache, weight gain, oily skin, muscle spasm, altered fat metabolism, rashes, deepening of the voice, additional hair growth and mood changes.

Gonadotrophin-releasing hormone analogues

Substances called gonadotrophin-releasing hormone analogues (GnRH agonists, also known as luteinising hormone releasing hormone agonists or LHRH agonists) are among the most widely used medical therapies for excessive menstrual bleeding. They cause a marked drop in oestrogen levels by inducing a temporary menopause. Women have fewer or no periods, their fibroids tend to shrink and the endometrium thins. Once the treatment stops, the oestrogen levels rise and menstrual bleeding rapidly returns. In spite of this, a significant number of women claim to experience a 'carry over' benefit from the treatment and many are able to avoid hysterectomy, particularly if they started treatment when their menopause was imminent.

Adverse effects of these drugs, which occur to some extent in the majority of women treated, include hot flushes, vaginal dryness, mood changes, headache, altered breast size and reduced interest in sex. Long-term use can reduce bone strength (increasing the risk of osteoporosis and subsequent fractures) and can detrimentally affect the composition of fats in the blood (increasing the risk of heart disease). Before any woman starts on GnRH agonist therapy, her risk factors for osteoporosis — including family history, slight build, heavy smoking, low dietary calcium intake and chronic lack of exercise — should be assessed carefully. The data currently available suggest that bone loss may be only partially reversed when the therapy stops.

Treatment with GnRH agonists is often used prior to myomectomy (see later this chapter) in women with large fibroids because most surgeons prefer to remove small growths, believing the procedure will be less difficult and the results better. In a small number of women with fibroids the unexpected happens and heavy bleeding requiring blood transfusion follows GnRH agonist use.

The recommended duration of therapy is six months, as safety data are not available for longer treatment. Any woman who takes GnRH agonists beyond this sort of time frame is usually advised to take low dose hormone therapy that includes both oestrogen and progestogen. This helps relieve the previously mentioned menopausal symptoms and helps minimise calcium loss from the bones.

Drug and non-drug treatments for painful periods

In severe cases of primary dysmenorrhoea (painful periods, see chapter 2) the pain can be stopped by suppressing ovulation. Drugs such as the contraceptive pill or NSAIDs with anti-prostaglandin activity (see earlier this chapter) may be useful.

Painkillers are widely used to deal with this pain and a variety of non-drug approaches may also help. Weekly acupuncture has been shown to ease painful periods in 90% of women, with a 41% reduction in the use of painkillers.[2] This approach may be attractive to women who want to handle their menstrual pain without medication, either because it is no longer effective or because of unacceptable side-effects. There is also evidence that lifestyle changes such as stopping smoking can reduce menstrual pain. Women treated non-surgically for painful periods report increased physical activity levels a year after starting treatment, but the majority are negative about the prospect of continuing on with their non-surgical efforts at pain relief.

Treatments for PMS and menopausal symptoms

Drug therapies

The contraceptive pill, transdermal oestradiol (Estraderm patch) and progesterone are drugs sometimes used to treat PMS, a condition whose cause is obscure. The thinking behind the use of these drug therapies is that if there is a hormone imbalance underlying PMS, it may be rectified by appropriate hormonal supplementation. Studies of the effectiveness of these treatments give inconclusive results, a possible reason being that PMS is an umbrella term for several different disorders which may reflect different hormonal disturbances.

Psychological therapies

The use of psychological therapies to treat PMS, various types of depression and menopausal symptoms such as hot flushes is based on the view that mental processes can play a significant role in the development and maintenance of these conditions and symptoms. Therapists treating women with PMS have used coping-skills therapies to alleviate the condition.[3] These therapies have three main components. First, individuals are taught to examine their ways of responding to stressful situations. The second phase involves rehearsing new coping strategies that are based on a major re-think of the way they respond to stressful life events. In the third phase, women test their coping responses in the stressful situations that previously gave rise to their PMS and depression. Training programs, which sometimes incorporate relaxation skills, generally involve ninety-minute sessions once a week for eight to ten weeks.

In the case of Nina, aged forty, who had had unrelenting PMS for much of her adult life, coping-skills therapy helped her to identify cues associated with her irritability and feelings of tension and fatigue. She became aware that her approaching menstrual period generated feelings of having to 'get things done' in anticipation of her 'bad days' when even small things required an enormous effort. Instead of allowing these feelings to dominate her activities, causing overloading and a self-fulfilling exhaustion, she trained herself to develop a plan of action. 'Don't concern yourself about the bad days, just about what you have to do today,' she told herself. 'Keep the focus on the present.' After several months she considered her PMS to be much less of a problem.

Biofeedback training

Some women have found training in biofeedback, meditation and relaxation to be valuable in their efforts to control hot flushes. Using biofeedback techniques individuals learn to manipulate body functions usually regarded as independent of conscious control. In a typical biofeedback training program, an instrument capable of measuring blood vessel opening or closure is attached to the skin of a woman with a hot flush problem. The machine transforms the feedback from the instrument into a beep or flashing light so that awareness of the approach of a hot flush grows and methods of short-circuiting the flush can be explored.

Herbal therapies and nutritional supplementation

Interest in herbal and other alternative therapies (also called complementary therapies) has escalated in many industrialised countries since the 1970s. The reasons are complex but probably include an increasing scepticism about science, and a public that is less willing to accept the truth of statements by 'experts' including medical practitioners. Periodic national health surveys in Australia from 1977 to 1990 show progressive increases in the number of consultations with alternative therapists. At the same time numerous doctors and others involved in health care have highlighted problems with medical knowledge, for example the limited perspective which drives certain treatment approaches. Recognition that other perspectives may have something valuable to offer is evident among practitioners and trainees of mainstream Western medicine.

A recent survey in Britain showed that 80% of doctors want to include some form of alternative medicine in their practices; and a recent study of Australian fourth year medical students found that an overwhelming majority of 92% were keen to study alternative medicine as part of their degree.[4] The students were most interested in meditation, nutritional medicine, acupuncture, naturopathy, Chinese herbal medicine, homeopathy, hypnosis and the ancient Indian treatment, ayurvedic.

A criticism commonly made about alternative therapies is the lack of solid scientific evidence about their effectiveness and safety, a problem compounded by the lack of quality control in the manufacture of some substances. These therapies have, for the most part, not been submitted to the sort of evaluation of efficacy (double-blind trial) required in recent decades for drugs used in orthodox medicine. While some alternative therapies have stood the test of time, having been used for centuries in some countries, careful long-term studies of risks and benefits tend to be lacking or only recently initiated. Ironically, while orthodox medicine is becoming more open to alternative approaches, alternative medicine is now being submitted to increased scientific scrutiny. As evidence of this, the manufacture of herbal medicines in Australia has been governed by an act of federal parliament since 1993 and the Australian government recently established a Traditional Medicine Evaluation Committee within the federal Department of Health.

Many of the alternative therapies share a common philosophy that life-giving energies and substances help maintain the human body in good health and balance. Ill-health is regarded as the result of a loss of balance caused by a sub-optimal lifestyle or an accumulation of toxic substances, including the products of infectious disease. To correct disturbances to the body's balance, or to maintain the existing equilibrium, the alternative therapies adopt a holistic treatment approach that emphasises the patient rather than a problem organism or toxin. The focus is on an individual's ability to overcome disease with the help of substances that clean and strengthen the body, rather than on the disease-destroying abilities of particular pharmaceuticals.

It is sometimes assumed that because herbal products and nutritional supplements are of natural origins they are therefore free from serious ill-effects. Unfortunately this is not always so. All herbal and nutritional supplements should be used cautiously and monitored regularly by a skilled practitioner, because adverse effects can occur — just as they can with orthodox medicines.

One of the most important herbs used by herbal therapists for the treatment of hormone problems in women is *Vitex agnus castus* (also called Chaste Berry or Monk's Pepper). It is derived from the ripe berries of a Mediterranean shrub but the chemical constituents said to be responsible for its actions in balancing the menstrual cycle have not been defined. Treatment is long-term over many months using doses of about 2 to 3 ml of a 1:5 tincture a day (this means that 5 ml of the final preparation is equivalent to one gram of the dried herb from which the preparation was made). It is common practice in England, and also recommended by German manufacturers, to take *Vitex* in a single dose each morning before breakfast throughout the cycle. Prolonged use of high doses is not advisable, but a course of six months treatment without a break is said to be necessary for full and lasting improvement. Headache is an occasional side-effect.

The first major clinical studies on *Vitex*, published in the 1950s, claimed significant improvements in over 60%

of women treated for heavy or frequent bleeding.[5] The average duration of bleeding was said to decrease from eight to five days. An English herbalist, Janet Hicks, claims that heavy and prolonged bleeding is best tackled by combining *Vitex* with muscle relaxants. When women experience symptoms of PMS such as irritability, and menopausal symptoms like hot flushes, she suggests they take *Vitex*. Then, as the PMS disappears, another herb, *Chamaelirium luteum* (Holonias), is recommended. Mrs Hicks considers *Vitex* unsuitable for post-menopausal women and women of any age using hormones such as the Pill, hormone therapy or danazol.

A host of other herbal and nutritional therapies are also in widespread use. The seeds of the horsechestnut are said to be helpful for painful periods; ginseng, motherwort, lime blossom, *Cimicifuga racemosa*, vitamin E and evening primrose oil tablets are all capable of affecting hot flushes; and vitamin B_6 (pyridoxine), evening primrose oil and *Anemone pulsatilla* can apparently alleviate PMS in some women. At least part of the benefit of these treatments lies in a placebo effect, that is, an effect that is just the same when a harmless substance like a sugar pill is substituted for the substance being tested. This effect is not well-understood but it is well-documented with both orthodox and alternative medicines. It is said to occur in a third or more patients when most treatments are tested.[6] It may be that people seek help from health practitioners when their symptoms are at their worst and, when they start to feel better, they put it down to the treatment — although they may have felt better in the same time regardless of whether or not they received treatment. Another possible explanation is that the brain releases chemicals that, for example, suppress pain as a conditioned reflex to receiving a pharmaceutical or alternative medication.

An important nutritional supplement for many women with heavy or prolonged bleeding is iron tablets, which can help to relieve anaemia (see chapter 2) and associated fatigue. A study of 380 women in the US State of Maine, whose fibroids, abnormal bleeding and chronic pelvic pain were managed without surgery, found that about 6% of those with abnormal bleeding or fibroids had anaemia.[7] A comparison study also conducted in Maine found that 19% of women having hysterectomies for fibroids were anaemic.[8] A measurement of blood haemoglobin (the pigmented substance that gives red blood cells their colour and also carries oxygen through the body) will show whether anaemia is a problem. The iron most easily absorbed by the human body is found in lean meat (especially liver and kidneys), seafoods (especially oysters) and poultry. Less-easily absorbed iron is present in cereals, legumes, vegetables (especially green leafy varieties) and eggs.

The commonly held view that vitamin B_6 will cure symptoms of PMS has resulted in many women taking high doses of it (several hundred milligrams a day). Dosages above 25 mg a day are inadvisable as they can lead to damage of the nerve endings in the fingers and toes, as well as dependence. Rather than taking high doses of B_6, it is worth considering boosting your intake of foods rich in this vitamin such as bananas, lentils, avocado, fish, eggs, turkey, chicken, tuna, salmon, walnuts and lean meat.

Treatments for endometriosis

Despite a considerable amount of energy, ingenuity and research in recent years, the cause of endometriosis remains shrouded in mystery. This has undoubtedly slowed progress in developing effective treatments.

Drug therapies

Drugs such as danazol, progestogens and GnRH agonists are capable of shrinking endometriosis tissue. They work by blocking the action of oestrogen which seems to be an essential ingredient in endometriosis growth. While these drug therapies are not capable of eliminating severe endometriosis, they are often used in the lead-up to surgical, electrical or laser treatment in the hope of making the removal of endometriosis tissue safer and more effective. Many doctors prefer not to prescribe danazol, progestogens at low dose, or GnRH agonists for longer than six months because of side-effects such as weight gain, breast tenderness, depression, nausea and hot flushes. There is also little information about the effects of long-term usage but what we do know gives cause for concern. For example, danazol has adverse effects on blood fats and GnRH agonists cause loss of calcium from bones. For some women, high daily doses of progestogens cause few problems and this therapy may be recommended when endometriosis recurs after other attempts to remove it.

Surgical treatments

Excisional surgery for endometriosis means cutting and removing or destroying endometriosis tissue wherever it lies in the pelvis. The surgery can be performed in a traditional manner through a large, open abdominal incision about 13 cm wide (open excisional surgery at laparotomy) or during a laparoscopy, in which the inside of the pelvis is viewed through a laparoscope, a tubular instrument with a light at one end and an eyepiece at the other, which is used to 'spotlight' internal organs (figure 7).

If surgery is to be performed in the latter manner, a woman is anaesthetised for laparoscopy (usually a gen-

Figure 7   The two most common laparoscopic procedures for removal of endometriosis growth

a Laser or diathermy

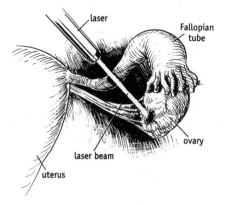

b Excision

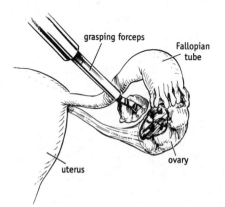

eral anaesthetic) and then several small incisions (up to 1 cm each) are made in her abdominal wall. A needle inserted through one of these incisions is used to introduce carbon dioxide or nitrous oxide gas into the abdomen. The gas separates the organs from each other so that the doctor can gain a clear view. The gas also expands the abdomen, making the woman look about six months pregnant — but only until the end of the procedure when she regains her normal shape. Meanwhile, the laparoscope and any other instruments needed to cut out endometriosis tissue are introduced through the other incisions. For instance, a laser (for laser vaporisation) or an electrocoagulation device (for diathermy) may be inserted. After laparoscopic excision of endometriosis tissue, the laparoscope and other instruments are removed, the gas is allowed to escape and all incisions are closed with a suture or two. The American College of Obstetricians and Gynecologists rates electrocoagulation and laser treatment as equally good options for destroying endometriosis at laparoscopy.

Long-term information about the efficacy of surgical approaches in removing endometriosis and reducing its symptoms suggests that they may be about twice as effective as drug therapies. Success rates are around 80% with surgery and about 40% with drug treatments. Whichever technique is under consideration, women should be aware of the risks of these procedures. General anaesthesia can cause nausea, vomiting and impaired concentration for some time after surgery. The potential complications of excisional surgery with or without laparoscopy include bleeding, infection, damage to internal organs and the resultant need for another operation to repair any damage. Following laparoscopy, some discomfort is normal for a few days. Pain in the shoulders, neck or abdomen may occur if the gas used within the abdominal cavity is not removed completely. Very occasionally, a life-threatening air embolism occurs, in which a bubble of air enters the bloodstream and produces an obstruction in the heart or elsewhere.

Curettage and hysteroscopy

When it comes to disorders affecting the uterus, the procedure known as dilatation and curettage (D and C) is grossly overused. There is now ample research indicating it has significant shortcomings, yet it continues to be carried out both to provide samples of tissue for further investigation and as a 'treatment' for women with menstrual irregularities. In fact, its ability to provide useful samples for diagnostic purposes is quite limited; and when used for treatment purposes it is very disappointing, reducing menstrual flow for only one cycle in most women. In 1991–92 in New South Wales alone, more than 35 000 D and Cs were performed, suggesting that the annual figure for this procedure in Australia probably exceeds 100 000.

The D and C technique is usually carried out under a general anaesthetic in a day hospital or general hospital setting. During dilatation, the cervix is gently stretched open by inserting progressively larger instruments. This is followed by a curette in which the endometrium is gently scraped away using an elongated instrument with a scoop attachment.

An alternative diagnostic procedure that can be used when a detailed patient history, examination and laboratory tests have failed to reveal the cause of abnormal bleeding is hysteroscopy. A hysteroscope is basically a tubular instrument with a light at one end and an optical system for transmitting an image to a display monitor. It is inserted through the vagina and cervix to observe the inside of the uterus. After obtaining ultrasound images of the uterus and introducing gas to separate the pelvic organs, the cervical canal is gently stretched to allow the hysteroscope to pass into it. It is then possible to get a good view of the uterus in about 80% of patients. (In the remaining patients, the view may be obscured by heavy bleeding.) Of women with menstrual irregularities in whom the uterus can be observed, more than 60% have no apparent uterine abnormality. These women are spared a diagnostic curettage. The others may have fibroids, polyps, endometriosis, pre-cancerous changes or endometrial cancer. If any area of abnormality is identified, a sample can be removed, checked by a pathologist and, in many cases, destroyed on the spot by an instrument inserted through the hysteroscope.

Hysteroscopy is thus a useful diagnostic test which can be used as the basis for treatment. It can be carried out without hospital admission or general anaesthesia, a considerable benefit in the eyes of many women (particularly those who are elderly and have multiple medical problems). A study by the University of Adelaide and the Royal Adelaide Hospital suggests that Australia's health budget could be reduced by at least $30 million a year if outpatient hysteroscopy (also called office hysteroscopy) was adopted instead of performing D and C procedures in day surgery units.[9] This 1994 study quoted the cost of a hysteroscopy at about $100, while a D and C cost over $500 when carried out in a day surgery unit and over $1000 if an operating theatre and overnight stay were required.

Serious complications such as bowel perforation occur in less than 1% of patients having a hysteroscopy, but about 70% experience the discomfort of menstrual-type pain, sensations of dizziness, tremor, shoulder tip pain or nausea, which is often followed by vomiting. If doctors explain possible side-effects before the procedure starts, this can help to reduce anxiety in patients when they occur. As increasing numbers of gynaecologists become familiar with the technique of hysteroscopy, it is hoped that D and C will be used more selectively.

Endometrial ablation and resection

Various procedures have been developed in recent years which aim to destroy the endometrium in women experiencing excessive bleeding that is resistant to control by drug therapy. The heavy or prolonged bleeding may be caused by fibroids, adenomyosis, post-menopausal hormone therapy or drugs designed to thin the blood (anticoagulant therapy). These procedures do not appear to be helpful in relieving pain associated with menstruation.

The destruction process is carried out using a hystero-scope, an instrument described previously in this chapter. A fibre optic camera threaded through the hysteroscope records the view which is seen by the surgeon on a video screen. The surgeon, who needs good hand–eye coordination, watches the image on the screen, enabling him or her to guide various instruments in the confined space of the uterus. These instruments can include a ball heated by an electrical current (called a rollerball), an electrically heated wire loop (called a resectoscope) or a laser. The procedure is referred to as an endometrial resection when the electrically heated ball or wire loop is used to produce electrocoagulation (also called diathermy) of the endometrium, and an

Figure 8 Endometrial resection and ablation techniques

a Endometrial resection using the resectoscope with a rollerball attached

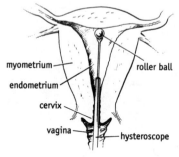

b Endometrial resection using a resectoscope loop

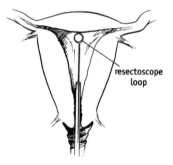

c Endometrial ablation using a laser

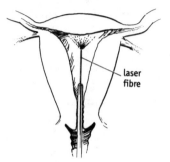

endometrial ablation when heat from a laser is used. The rollerball method of endometrial resection destroys the endometrium by rolling the coagulating ball over it like a paint roller, the electrocoagulation loop removes or ploughs several furrows in it, and the laser vaporises it (figure 8). In the case of endometrial ablation, light from the laser passes down an optical fibre inserted into the hysteroscope and the surgeon moves the tip of the laser to draw a fine beam of light across the endometrium. In radiofrequency ablation, high energy radio frequency waves are applied to the endometrium instead of the high energy laser beam. A thermal method of removing the endometrium which involves passing hot water into the uterus is also being developed. Early studies suggest it is just as effective as methods using laser or electrocoagulation and may have advantages over them in terms of safety.

Comparisons of the resectoscope and the laser suggest that the former is cheaper, more readily available in hospitals, faster to use, takes less time for doctors to become competent with, is more robust and results in fewer complications. As the techniques alter, however, claims to superiority may be short-lived. A study comparing the newer ablation technique of radiofrequency with endometrial resection claims the former is simpler to perform, less time-consuming and possibly safer. However its cost is higher and the success rate is comparable.

Women having these procedures can receive either a general anaesthetic or a local anaesthetic with light sedation, although, for the laser treatment, a general anaesthetic is currently the norm. A few women bleed heavily immediately after the operation; but, for most, light post-operative bleeding gradually turns into a light discharge that disappears completely over about four to six weeks. Periods may continue, and in most cases they are light. Most women are in hospital for a day or overnight, and many have resumed work within a week or two. A year after an endometrial ablation or resection, about 85% of women report having reduced their use of sanitary pads or tampons by more than half; some have no bleeding at all, while for others heavy bleeding is still a problem. Looked at over a ten-year time frame, there is still a dearth of data.

The endometrium is well-known for its regenerative powers, provoking speculation that removing the endometrium is just 'one more operation of doubtful value' that women are being encouraged to have. One study of more than 400 women who had endometrial resections for fibroids, endometriosis or adenomyosis found that about 20% developed a recurrence of heavy bleeding within four years, in some cases within a few months of the procedure.[10] Some of these women chose to have the procedure repeated but, after a second try, about 40% of this group were still having bleeding problems. Overall, about one in every eight women who had an endometrial resection ended up having a hysterectomy within four years. Women who had a repeat resection were even more likely to resort to hysterectomy, with more than one in three such women eventually having the operation.

Endometrial resection and ablation were introduced in the late 1970s in the US and are now routine procedures in many hospitals. Many tens of thousands of the procedures are performed worldwide each year. The speed with which the techniques have been taken up by medicine has surprised and shocked many people who say that fundamental questions about their safety, effectiveness and long-term consequences have not been resolved.

Information about the suitability of different groups of women for these procedures is scant. The available evidence suggests that women with a normal sized uterus or those who are on post-menopausal hormone therapy tend to do well, while those with a uterus that is enlarged by fibroids, markedly retroverted (tilted backwards) or who have severe adenomyosis or endometriosis may be unsuitable. Women at risk from a general anaesthetic — such as women who are very overweight, and those with chronic liver, kidney or heart disease — may prefer the option of an endometrial resection or ablation because it is possible to do either under local anaesthesia. Selection of women most likely to benefit from the procedure is extremely important and obviously influences the outcome for them. In this regard, the visualisation of the reproductive organs using ultrasound can be especially helpful in deciding the appropriateness of these procedures.

Endometrial ablation and resection are not risk-free but complication rates appear to be lower than for hysterectomy. Complications include infection (affecting one in every 100 women having the procedure), bleeding (less than one per 100), damage to the bowel or other pelvic structures including major blood vessels (one to two women in every 100 suffers a perforated organ or blood vessel), and fluid overload (one to two per 100).[11] Studies to date suggest that about two women in every 10 000 having the procedure die as a result of it. By way of comparison, the death rate for abdominal hysterectomy in fit women of reproductive age is between one and six deaths per 10 000. Because the technique is relatively new, long-term effects are not known.

Studies comparing endometrial ablation or resection with abdominal hysterectomy suggest that the former offers benefits in terms of post-operative pain, hospital stay, convalescence, risks and financial cost. Satisfaction among women after having a hysterectomy seems, however, to be significantly higher than among those whose endometrium has been removed (94% compared with 85% in the Maine studies referred to earlier in this chapter). This may reflect the 'failure rate' of endometrial resection or ablation — women who are hoping that their bleeding problems will resolve are likely to feel dissatisfied with the procedure even if they have been warned in advance that it is not a universal success. It might also suggest that the procedure is being oversold or that patient selection is not as good as it could be.

Endometrial resection or ablation is probably the treatment of choice for women who want short-term relief from bleeding problems, and who are keen to minimise the risk of complications, the financial cost of treatment and the time off work. Hysterectomy is probably a better option for women wanting certain and complete relief from bleeding problems. It may also be the preferred option of women with an increased risk of endometrial cancer, which includes women with a family history of the disease, those with polycystic ovaries, those who use oestrogen on its own without added progestogen, and women who are obese or who have diabetes.

Cost is probably one of the major reasons for the rapid uptake of these procedures. In a recent Australian survey the cost of endometrial resection was estimated at $1500, which is less than half the cost of an abdominal hysterectomy.[12] The cost of endometrial ablation was about $2200 to $2500 depending on the type of equipment used. The relative cost advantage of these techniques over hysterectomy may, however, be eroded if re-treatment and later hysterectomies occur more often than has been reported to date.

A recent article in the popular science magazine *New Scientist* emphasised that doctors who perform endometrial resection or ablation are on a learning curve.[13] To produce good results they need to be experienced in the technique of hysteroscopy and to have served an apprenticeship in hysteroscopic surgery under a knowledgable supervisor. 'Reports from surgeons suggest that serious complications are most likely to occur while the gynaecologist is still on the 'learning curve', which can last for anything between 10 and 80 operations,' the article said. 'Studies have shown that 50% of perforations of the womb take place in the first five operations a surgeon carries out.' It is important to find out where on this learning curve your surgeon is before agreeing to any procedure. Refer to chapter 5 for a discussion of how to do this.

Myomectomy for fibroids

Myomectomy is the surgical removal of one or more fibroids from the uterus with the aim of providing relief from prolonged or heavy bleeding. It is an option worth considering for women who have not finished their families and who therefore want their uterus intact to preserve their fertility. Pregnancy rates of 40–59% following myomectomy have been reported. It is, however, a difficult operation which is more likely than hysterectomy to cause blood loss requiring transfusion and postoperative ill-health. For these reasons, women with fibroids are five times more likely to have a hysterectomy than a myomectomy.

In most women, myomectomy initially relieves bleeding symptoms. But, ten years after the operation, 20–30% have returned to their doctors with a recurrence of their earlier problems. The reasons for this recurrence rate are as uncertain as the reasons for the development of fibroids in the first place. There is some evidence to suggest that recurrence rates are higher when multiple fibroids are present or the initial fibroid removal is incomplete. The latter suggestion is, however, hotly disputed; and there is also support for the view that it is only necessary to remove that part of the fibroid protruding from the wall of the uterus to obtain long-lasting relief from heavy bleeding. It has also been suggested that some women have an inherited tendency to develop fibroids and that this has a big influence on the recurrence rate.

Abdominal or open myomectomy, where the operation is performed through a large (approximately 13 cm) incision, has been the procedure used for many years. Recently, several new approaches have been devised which make use of a hysteroscope inserted through the vagina (hysteroscopic myomectomy), or a laparoscope inserted in the abdomen (laparoscopic myomectomy). These procedures avoid the need for large abdominal incisions. (Similar techniques may be used to remove adenomyosis, a condition that is closely related to fibroids.) A vaginal ultrasound showing the position and size of fibroids is helpful in deciding which of the above approaches is advisable.

Open myomectomy is performed more often in Australia than hysteroscopic or laparoscopic myomectomy. Likely explanations for this include the suitability of open myomectomy for the removal of large fibroids and for the removal of fibroids from sites where they are often found, such as the outer wall of the uterus. Open myomectomy is also a more entrenched procedure than either hysteroscopic or laparoscopic fibroid removal.

Fibroids up to 8 cm in size can also be made smaller or destroyed using laser techniques or electrocoagulation. Some doctors are becoming skilled in these techniques, making them increasingly suitable alternatives to myomectomy, particularly for women with heavy periods.

Whichever method is employed, the procedure should be conducted in a well-equipped clinic or hospital under general anaesthesia. During the removal of fibroids it is important that the surgeon minimises blood loss and the inadvertent formation of adhesions, and that he or she skilfully reconstructs the uterus. Some blood loss is inevitable as the uterus is particularly well supplied with arteries and veins. It is usual for surgeons to clamp blood vessels or to inject chemicals that decrease the flow of blood to certain areas of the uterus. Particular types and locations of incisions also help minimise blood loss during myomectomy as does the use of laser surgery or diathermy in experienced hands. In some cases, doctors may remove the endometrium at the same time as performing a myomectomy. (See descriptions of endometrial resection and ablation earlier in this chapter.)

The formation of adhesions — a risk of any abdominal surgery — must be avoided if possible because of the associated pain and interference with normal organ function. Tissues that were never meant to be joined can become attached to each other and problems like chronic pelvic pain and infertility may result. To minimise the chances of adhesions forming, tissues must be handled gently, appropriate irrigation solutions or an adhesion barrier used within the abdomen, and blood loss minimised. The extra cost to the patient of taking these precautions is less than $150, a small price to pay for the prevention of potentially serious problems. The use of laser techniques and diathermy also appears to reduce the risk of adhesion formation. Reconstruction of the uterus after removal of fibroids requires skill and care. Recent research suggests that when sutures are avoided during myomectomy, adhesions are less likely to develop. On the other hand, the absence of sutures may lead to weakness of the uterus.

An occasional serious complication of hysteroscopic myomectomy is perforation of the uterus. It may occur if the surgeon cuts deeply into the wall of the uterus to remove parts of an embedded fibroid. To minimise the risk of this happening, some doctors simultaneously perform a laparoscopy, a procedure in which a small incision in the abdomen is used as a porthole to enable visual inspection of the pelvic organs, including the outside wall of the uterus. Others think this is of doubtful value. Most women return home within one to three days of a hysteroscopic or laparoscopic myomectomy and it is usual for surgeons to check on each patient's progress about six weeks later.

For open myomectomy, the pattern of post-operative illness and time to full recovery is similar to that for abdominal hysterectomy. That is, the average length of hospital stay is four to seven days, pain persists for several weeks and full recovery may take several months.

Women having a hysteroscopic or laparoscopic myomectomy experience less pain and a shorter convalescence (by about two to four weeks) than those having either open myomectomy or abdominal hysterectomy. The cost of these procedures in Australia is considerably less, in the short-term at least, than the cost of an open myomectomy (around $1500 for hysteroscopic myomectomy and $2200 for a laparoscopic myomectomy compared to $3825 for an open myomectomy).[14] Because of the relatively recent introduction of hysteroscopic and laparoscopic techniques to perform myomectomy, it will be some time before we know the extent to which fibroid recurrence and complications alter these costings.

four

Hysterectomy procedures

Hysterectomy has long been the most commonly used method of surgically treating women for gynaecological problems such as excessive menstrual bleeding and chronic pelvic pain. Recent years have seen both numerous changes in the way that hysterectomies are performed, and a variety of new techniques (described in the previous chapter) that are challenging its dominance.

Types of hysterectomy

The term 'hysterectomy' originates from the Greek words hystera, meaning uterus, and ektome, to cut out. The earliest hysterectomies on record were performed about 1600 years ago in Greece and, despite high death rates until last century, the procedure is still carried out. There are four basic types of hysterectomy.

Total hysterectomy

A total hysterectomy refers to removal of the entire uterus including the cervix, together with its supporting ligaments, while leaving the Fallopian tubes and ovaries in place (figure 9).

Total hysterectomy with salpingo-oophorectomy

A total hysterectomy with salpingo-oophorectomy entails removing the uterus with cervix and support ligaments, together with one or both sets of ovaries and Fallopian tubes. If both sets are removed the operation is called a total hysterectomy with bilateral salpingo-oophorectomy (figure 10).

Subtotal (or partial) hysterectomy

A subtotal (or partial) hysterectomy involves removal of the upper two-thirds of the uterus only. The cervix is left intact, along with the Fallopian tubes and ovaries (figure 11).

Radical or Wertheim's hysterectomy

A radical hysterectomy means that the surgeon removes the entire uterus including cervix and support structures, both ovaries, Fallopian tubes, nearby lymph nodes, and the upper portion of the vagina (figure 12).

In some women, for example a patient with cancer that has infiltrated several reproductive organs, there may be no option but a radical hysterectomy. In other circumstances there may be more flexibility about the amount of tissue taken.

By the time Robyn turned thirty-seven her medical history included a myomectomy and an endometrial resection. Both procedures were undertaken to control heavy bleeding due to fibroids, but neither provided lasting relief. She had decided to accept the advice of her gynaecologist and have a hysterectomy, but was uncertain which sort would be most appropriate. The doctor proposed removing her ovaries and Fallopian tubes,

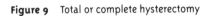

Figure 9   Total or complete hysterectomy

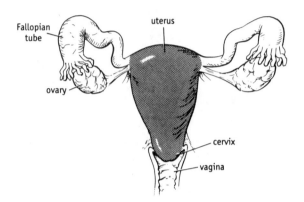

Figure 10   Total hysterectomy with bilateral salpingo-oophorectomy

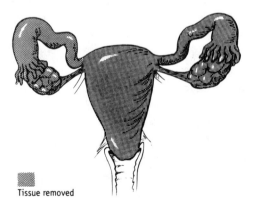

Figure 11   Subtotal or partial hysterectomy

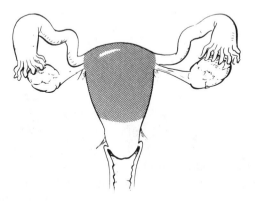

Figure 12   Radical or Wertheim's hysterectomy

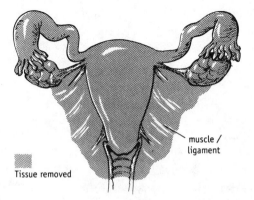

muscle /
ligament

Tissue removed

along with her uterus, because of the possibility that ovarian cancer could develop some time in the future. This form of cancer tends to evade detection until it is advanced; treatment prospects are then poor. Robyn asked about the short- and long-term implications of ovary removal at her age and was told that her menopause would occur earlier than expected. Acute menopausal symptoms such as hot flushes and vaginal dryness were likely to accompany an early menopause, and hormone therapy would then be advisable. Long-term implications included an elevated risk of osteoporosis and heart disease. Even if the ovaries were left it was possible that she might experience a somewhat earlier than expected menopause, although this was by no means certain. As Robyn's family had a tendency for heart disease, but not for ovarian cancer, she declined to have a total hysterectomy with bilateral salpingo-oophorectomy. Instead, a total hysterectomy was performed, and care was taken to preserve her ovaries intact.

There may also be some flexibility when it comes to the question of removal of the cervix. Women who have asked doctors about the implications of losing their cervix and the upper part of their vagina have received varied responses according to whether they were pre- or post-menopausal. Pre-menopausal women whose ovaries are to remain may be told to expect a reduced amount of lubricative cervical mucus around the time of the month that they ovulate. This might be one factor contributing to reduced sexual satisfaction for them and their sexual partners. At other times of the month when the output of cervical mucus is minimal, the impact of cervical secretions on sexual satisfaction would be negligible. Although recent studies do not show a reduction in vaginal size after the cervix has been removed, the absence of the cervix itself might be expected to alter the sensations experienced during intercourse. For post-menopausal women loss of the cervix would not affect lubrication, but its absence might alter sexual satisfaction for one or both partners if tapping it during intercourse was important for orgasm. On the other hand, removal of the cervix might be seen to have convenience value for some women as it would do away with the need for repeated Pap smears. It has become increasingly common to offer women the option of preservation of the ovaries and cervix and upper part of the vagina during hysterectomy.

Further ways of classifying hysterectomy

Surgeons gain access to, and remove, one or more of the reproductive organs in a number of ways. This is the basis for another method of classifying hysterectomy.

Abdominal hysterectomy

If access is gained via an incision in the abdomen, the operation is called an abdominal hysterectomy. This is usually performed when:

- one or both ovaries are to be removed
- there are large fibroids, endometriosis, pelvic inflammatory disease or tough adhesions surrounding the intestines
- the surgeon wants to examine by touch or inspect the abdominal organs because of suspicious symptoms
- the surgery is likely to be prolonged because, for example, the woman is obese.

The incision in the abdomen can be either vertical (an 'up and down' cut) or horizontal ('transverse'), and is about 13 cm in length. If the incision is horizontal, it is usually possible to minimise the visibility of any permanent scar by cutting near or below the pubic hairline (the so-called 'bikini cut') or along the line of a previous Caesarean scar. You should discuss the position of any scar before the operation to ensure your surgeon knows your views on this (figure 13).

Whatever type of hysterectomy is going to be performed, a pre-surgery ultrasound is useful as it can help decide which type of operation is likely to be most suitable, and it means the woman and the surgeon are better prepared for what lies ahead. It is reasonable for a woman to request an ultrasound if any form of hysterectomy is proposed.

Vaginal hysterectomy

If the reproductive organs are accessed through the vagina, the operation is called a vaginal hysterectomy (figure 14). This approach may be considered when:
- a woman has a prolapse and her uterus, bowel or bladder has already started to intrude into her vagina
- there are fibroids that are small enough to enable the uterus to be pulled down and out through the vagina
- the ovaries are to be left intact.

Vaginal hysterectomy is unsuitable when the uterus is very large or contains one or more sizeable fibroids. It is more difficult to perform than abdominal hysterectomy and should always begin and end with a laparoscopic inspection of the pelvis. This helps ensure that any abnormalities, such as ovarian cysts, are identified prior to surgery and alerts the surgeon to any bleeding that has occurred during the operation. Bleeding must be contained or the patient will form large blood clots in the pelvis which may lead to adhesion formation and

Figure 13 Incisions for three major types of hysterectomy

a Abdominal hysterectomy: 'up and down' or crossways cut of 6–12 cm

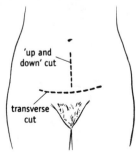

b Vaginal hysterectomy: incision in top of vagina of 5–6 cm

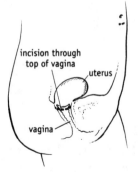

c Laparoscopically assisted hysterectomy: three to four small incisions of 0.5–1 cm

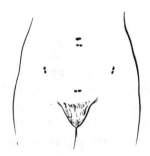

Figure 14 Laparoscopically assisted hysterectomy showing removal of the uterus through the vagina

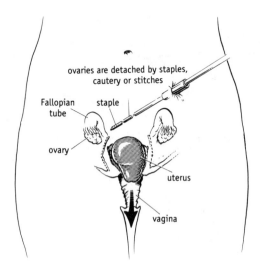

ovaries are detached by staples, cautery or stitches

Fallopian tube

staple

ovary

uterus

vagina

infection. Removal of any clots will involve another trip to the operating theatre and an extra two to three days in hospital.

The debate among doctors about the relative merits of abdominal and vaginal hysterectomies is ongoing. Proponents of the vaginal approach argue that it involves less post-operative pain, is less costly and requires a shorter hospital stay. Some research has suggested it may be safer than the abdominal approach, resulting in fewer deaths and a lower complication rate but analysis of Australian hospital data indicates that this is not necessarily so. Nevertheless it is argued that the vaginal approach could be used for most hysterectomies if appropriate training programs for doctors were available.

In contrast, doctors who favour the abdominal approach claim that the types of complications more likely to affect women having a vaginal hysterectomy are a cause for concern. They claim post-operative infection and large blood losses necessitating transfusions are more common with the vaginal approach; and they suggest that there is an increased risk of damage to other pelvic organs due to the confined space in which the surgery is performed. Repairing this damage entails further surgery. They also say that vaginal hysterectomy is more likely than abdominal hysterectomy to result in a vaginal prolapse, where the upper part of the vagina collapses inwards. The upshot is that at present in the US, UK and Australia, about 25% of hysterectomies are performed vaginally.

Laparoscopically assisted hysterectomy

In recent years, another technique has been developed that combines elements of both the abdominal and vaginal approaches. It entails using the laparoscope, described in chapter 3, to gain access to the abdomen through several small (about 1 cm) pelvic incisions. The laparoscopic view of the inside of the abdomen is transmitted to a video screen and the surgeon manipulates cutting, burning or laser instruments within the pelvis according to what is seen on the screen. Direct vision laparoscopy tends to be used only when perception of depth is unclear, otherwise all surgery is performed while watching the screen.

After detaching the uterus and any other organs to be removed with diathermy, and closing blood vessels and realigning tissues using staples or sutures, the surgeon makes an incision near the top of the vagina where it meets the cervix. The unwanted tissue is then extracted through the opening in the vagina. This technique is called laparoscopically assisted hysterectomy or laparovaginal hysterectomy. It has now been carried out on hundreds of women who would otherwise have had an abdominal hysterectomy. Laparoscopically assisted hysterectomy requires special equipment and a team of doctors and nurses skilled in gynaecological laparoscopy. It is considered to be suitable when:

- fibroids are of intermediate size
- endometriosis is a major reason for the surgery
- a reduced recovery period is important
- there is an early stage endometrial cancer and the ovaries are to be removed.

Margaret had a laparoscopically assisted hysterectomy instead of an abdominal or vaginal hysterectomy largely because of business pressures. A senior staff member of a company involved in a takeover bid, she was appreciative of the shorter hospital stay (one to four days instead of seven to ten days) and the reduced period of convalescence (one to four weeks instead of up to two or more months). After her convalescence it took her another few months to regain total well-being, but nevertheless she was able to contribute meaningfully at a critical time in her company's business operations.

There is some evidence that laparoscopically assisted hysterectomy has a lower complication rate than either vaginal or abdominal hysterectomy, although this claim has been disputed and the results of clinical trials are awaited with interest. The operation takes somewhat longer to carry out than the other types of hysterectomy (one to two hours on average, although the French have reduced their operating time to less than an hour, compared with thirty minutes to an hour for an abdominal hysterectomy) and requires more costly instruments.

Trends in types of hysterectomy

In Australia in the late 1980s, the vast majority of hysterectomy procedures were abdominal. By the early 1990s, however, vaginal procedures (including laparoscopically assisted hysterectomy) appeared to be gaining ground, increasing from 25 to 29% of all hysterectomies performed.[1] This is significant because the type of hysterectomy carried out influences the duration of and pain experienced after surgery, the time a woman spends in hospital and at home convalescing, and any postoperative complications she may experience.

Preparation for surgery

Any woman on the Pill should come off it a month before surgery, substituting a non-hormonal method of contraception, such as a condom or diaphragm in the meantime. Women who smoke should stop at least a week before a hysterectomy. They should also consider a permanent break from smoking as their risk of heart disease and osteoporosis is likely to increase as a result of the surgery, and smoking will increase this risk still further.

A GnRH agonist (see chapter 3) may be prescribed prior to surgery in a bid to reduce the size of any fibroids a woman may have. When this approach was systematically studied in 142 women, only half of whom received a GnRH agonist, the results were encouraging. The surgery was less likely to be difficult in the treated women who also experienced significantly less blood loss on average. It has been suggested that the beneficial effect of GnRH agonists is due partly to their ability to shrink fibroids and partly to their reduction of uterine blood flow.

Patient satisfaction with hysterectomy

The Maine Women's Health Study, one of the largest studies to date that has followed women through treatment for problems like heavy bleeding and chronic pelvic pain, presents a unique opportunity to compare hysterectomy with non-surgical therapies. In one part of the study over 350 women from the State of Maine, in the north-eastern United States, who had a hysterectomy were interviewed at the time of surgery and then three, six and twelve months later.[2] Most had been diagnosed as having fibroids, abnormal bleeding, chronic pelvic pain, endometriosis, a cancer, or prolapse. The peak age for hysterectomy in this group of mainly White women was the early forties. Another study was conducted at the same time for comparative purposes; it involved nearly 400 Maine women who had non-surgical treatment for fibroids, chronic pelvic pain and abnormal bleeding.[3] In general, the women who had hysterectomies had more severe symptoms than the non-surgical treatment group and their activities were more limited as a result.

The benefits of hysterectomy

The research team was surprised to find how strikingly beneficial hysterectomy was for symptom relief, and concluded that 'hysterectomy was associated with more marked improvement in symptoms and quality of life than nonsurgical therapy'. The women who had hysterectomies reported significant relief from bleeding problems, pelvic and back pain, pain during intercourse, abdominal swelling and urinary problems. Those who felt they benefited most from the surgery were those who had been most impaired by their symptoms. This impairment took the form of persistent discomfort or limitations on activity.

The study also found much lower rates of adverse effects of hysterectomy than expected. Earlier studies had reported problems with passing urine in 20–30% of women after hysterectomy, but the Maine study found this occurred in only 4%. Other studies have reported diminished sexual function in 15–30%, but although 7% of the Maine women reported being bothered by less interest in sex after their hysterectomy, only 1% reported less enjoyment of sexual activity, and the majority reported increased interest in, and enjoyment of, sex. Persistence of pelvic pain after hysterectomy has been reported to occur in 22% of women, but in Maine the figure was 5%. Importantly, 82% of women in the Maine study felt they had a choice about having the hysterectomy and, for most, six or more months elapsed between the decision to have surgery and the actual operation.

As a check on possible biases that might explain these sorts of findings, the Maine study authors looked at eligible patients who were not referred by their doctors to participate in the trial. They found that patients not in the study were more likely to feel that they had no choice about having a hysterectomy, and their mental health assessments were less positive than those of the women who had participated. It is possible that doctors selectively referred patients to the trial who were more involved in the treatment strategy and in a better state of mental health. It is also possible that improvements in surgical techniques and post-operative care are responsible for the more positive results that seem to be occurring. In the light of these uncertainties, the authors recommended that their study be repeated in other parts of the US.

Recent Australian research on the outcomes of hysterectomy has also found high levels of satisfaction among women having the operation, although this was tempered by the belief that some new symptoms had arisen which were caused by the surgery itself. Research by an Australian team from the University of Newcastle and Macquarie University, published in the *British Journal of Obstetrics and Gynaecology* in 1991, asked women who had had a hysterectomy between two and ten years earlier to describe the impact of their experience.[4] Of 175 women interviewed, 97% said the hysterectomy was worth the trouble and 88% said they would recommend a hysterectomy to others with similar problems, given their experience of it. The single most important benefit for 32% of the women was relief from heavy periods; for 25% it was relief from pain or painful periods; and for 4% it was improved emotional well-being.

An earlier Australian study, in which over 800 women who had had a hysterectomy (abdominal or vaginal) in New South Wales in 1976 or 1977 responded to a questionnaire, found that only about half were enthusiastic or very pleased that they had undergone the procedure.[5] About 11% were not satisfied with the outcome of the operation and almost 12% complained of poor doctor or nurse communication. Post-operative recovery was frequently longer than expected, with 70% requiring up to three months for a return to normal activities and 16%

more than six months. One impact that favourably impressed many women was sexual function, one-third indicating that this had improved after hysterectomy, while 3% reported a deterioration.

A recent English study compared patient satisfaction among nearly 200 women who were randomly assigned to abdominal hysterectomy or endometrial resection by diathermy.[6] It found a small but statistically significant difference in favour of satisfaction with hysterectomy four months after surgery. This was despite the fact that women having an endometrial resection experienced less post-operative ill-health than those who had a hysterectomy; a shorter hospital stay; and a swifter return to work, to normal daily activities and to sexual intercourse. The study, published in the *British Journal of Obstetrics and Gynaecology* in 1993, found that more than 10% of women who had an endometrial resection were dissatisfied at four months because of excessive or painful menstrual bleeding, bloating and breast tenderness. Other reasons for dissatisfaction included serious complications during the resection procedure, in particular perforation of the uterus during hysteroscopy. Based on the more positive response than expected to hysterectomy, the research team said longer-term comparative studies were necessary before endometrial resection was widely introduced. They also speculated that longer-term follow-up might show further improvements in satisfaction among women who had hysterectomies, but the reverse might be true for those who had an endometrial resection. The study stated that:

> The continuing requirement for cervical smears, uncertainty over future vaginal bleeding, risk of uterine and cervical cancer and need for a progestogen with menopausal oestrogen therapy may become important reasons for later

dissatisfaction with endometrial resection and may be more significant than the long-term complications of hysterectomy of premature ovarian failure and cardiovascular disease.

There is no doubt that many women feel like Caroline de Costa, quoted in chapter five, whose main emotions after hysterectomy were of enormous relief and genuine delight at the implications. 'I was now absolutely free of menstrual problems, would never have to worry about contraception again and could happily embark on hormone replacement therapy when I needed it without worrying about uterine bleeding.'[7]

The disadvantages of hysterectomy

Although a safer procedure than, for example, removal of the appendix, hysterectomy is not without risk.[8] For every 2000 abdominal hysterectomies performed, between one and four women die within a month of surgery (the variation in figures depends on which study is consulted). Death rates may be less for vaginal and laparoscopically assisted hysterectomies.

In addition, reports suggest that between 25 and 50% of all women who have a hysterectomy encounter one or more complications. In the case of abdominal hysterectomy, 1–3% of women experience a major complication such as significant post-operative bleeding, the formation of a blood clot in the lungs, or damage to the ureter, the bowel or the bladder, all of which may require further surgery. Vaginal prolapse and sexual problems may also occur with any type of hysterectomy because there is reduced support for the upper part of the vagina from other pelvic structures. To minimise this risk, the ligaments supporting the bladder, bowel and vagina are stitched together after the uterus is removed.

Other complications include infections of the surgical wound and urinary tract, weight gain, abdominal or back pain, constipation, fatigue and frequent urination. Some of these, for example urinary tract infections, usually clear quickly provided antibiotic therapy is administered promptly. In some women, however, they become a persistent source of unsettling symptoms requiring treatment. **For Rita, the biggest surprise following her hysterectomy was the kilos she suddenly gained. An enthusiast for keeping in shape, she couldn't understand why she had put on weight, given that she was just as careful about what she ate after her hysterectomy as before. 'My doctor thought it might have something to do with changes in my sex hormones, but when I asked about hormone replacement therapy he said this might cause even more weight gain.' Rita embarked on a vigorous schedule of physical activity which, at last report, had helped her weight to plateau.** She is not alone in experiencing this complication of hysterectomy. Some studies report that weight problems occur in nearly a quarter of women after the operation. It seems that women who want to maintain their weight at pre-hysterectomy levels need to be prepared to reduce their calorie intake somewhat in the two to six weeks after surgery in line with their reduced activity levels.

Psychological disturbances have been widely reported in women who have had hysterectomies, with depression, mood change, anxiety and irritability often cited. Other studies have, however, raised the possibility that it is not hysterectomy itself that triggers these disturbances. Rather, they may reflect psychological states which developed during the period of stress and ill-health preceding the operation.

For pre-menopausal women, hysterectomy may lead to an early menopause and distressing menopausal symptoms such as hot flushes and vaginal dryness if the ovaries are removed along with the uterus. This may also occur in women whose ovaries are saved, but less frequently, particularly if the surgeon who does the operation is skilful and experienced. An uncertain factor in all this is the state of the ovaries before surgery. It may be that women who resort to hysterectomy have a higher incidence of problems with their ovaries than women who do not, and that even if they were able to avoid surgery, their ovaries might not function particularly well. What can now be said with some certainty is that women who have had a hysterectomy are much more likely than average to embark on hormone therapy . The Melbourne Women's Midlife Health Project, which questioned 2000 randomly selected women aged forty-five to fifty-five years,[9] found that half the women who had both ovaries removed at the time of hysterectomy were on hormone therapy, as were a third who had a hysterectomy but retained their ovaries. In contrast about one in six women who had not had a hysterectomy was on hormone therapy. In a comparable group of US women, the rate was about the same in the surgical menopause group and significantly lower in the natural menopause group. Rates seem to vary widely across Western Europe, but there is not enough information to enable a valid comparison.

Other long-term complications, which stem in part from the early menopause that sometimes occurs after hysterectomy, are an increased risk of heart disease and of the bone thinning disorder, osteoporosis. In order to reduce these risks, as well as to resolve menopausal symptoms, hormone therapy containing oestrogen is often prescribed after a hysterectomy. Women may also be advised of the need for regular reviews of their blood fat levels and bone density and of the need to make lifestyle changes such as those discussed in chapter 7.

Weighing up the benefits and problems

Many women report a marked improvement in their symptoms after hysterectomy. Others experience a worsening of some symptoms, or the emergence of new symptoms that they attribute to the operation. The University of Newcastle/Macquarie University study mentioned earlier in this chapter found that while two-thirds of women considered that the symptoms they had before hysterectomy were improved by the operation, nearly as many women had symptoms which they thought were made worse or were caused by their hysterectomy. Participating women generally experienced less abdominal and back pain than before the operation, their incontinence improved, sex was less painful and they were less tired and tearful. However 29% were concerned about the development of hot flushes since their hysterectomy, 21% now had vaginal dryness and 17% had weight problems. Many also said they found the convalescence more difficult than they had expected, with pain a particular problem. Sizeable numbers would have liked more information about what was involved in recovering from hysterectomy before deciding on the operation, as well as more help in dealing with emotional problems associated with it and more information about alternative treatments. A small proportion thought they were worse off; 4% said the operation caused more problems than it solved and 7% that they would not have gone ahead had they fully understood what it entailed. Despite this, 96%

of the women said they were satisfied that they had had the right treatment, and 95% said they would make the same decision again if the circumstances were the same.

The Maine study of hysterectomy also reported on the advantages and disadvantages of the operation. Many of the women who took part experienced relief from symptoms — especially pelvic pain, urinary symptoms, fatigue, psychological symptoms and sexual problems — although once again some women experienced new problems after hysterectomy including hot flushes (13%), weight gain (12%), depression (8%) and lack of interest in sex (7%). Many of the symptoms women experience after hysterectomy seem to relate to a downturn in the function of their ovaries. If women are aware of this they can give consideration before surgery to the possibility that hysterectomy and hormone therapy may turn out to be a 'package', both components of which are necessary to achieve an improved quality of life.

It is difficult to reconcile the prevalence of new or unresolved symptoms following hysterectomy and the generally high levels of satisfaction with it. Obviously there are many aspects that each woman needs to explore before embarking on a major medical treatment like hysterectomy. This may be more easily said than done; it amounts to putting a value on removal of our present problems while trying to estimate what value we place on a range of future possibilities that may or may not occur. In other words, the symptoms of pelvic pain, difficult bleeding and fatigue that encourage many women to have a hysterectomy are in the 'here and now'. They make everyday living a chore, or worse, a nightmare. Furthermore many women who have hysterectomies have tried other treatments and found them wanting. In contrast, the outcome of hysterectomy is in the future. Every woman having the operation hopes it will relieve every symptom she has and create no new problems. Realistically, this may not occur. While one can comprehend in one's mind the fact that up to half of the women who have a hysterectomy experience some adverse effects, and that these may resolve quickly or have a negative impact on quality of life long-term, there is always the possibility that a particular individual will be fortunate and experience no down side. Perhaps women with an optimistic frame of mind are more likely to 'take the punt' on hysterectomy than those with a pessimistic bent. Making a decision that takes account of all the possibilities is more difficult.

Recuperation after hysterectomy

Information about recovery after hysterectomy is sometimes neglected in discussions between women and their doctors. Compared with the decision to have the operation and the demands of surgery, recovery may seem straightforward. Often, however, this does not prove to be the case.

The process of recovery from hysterectomy is extremely variable as illustrated by the experiences of Rosa and Denise, neither of whom had any postoperative complications. The day after her hysterectomy Rosa helped make beds in the hospital ward and, five days later, she was ready to leave. Within a few days she was doing all the housework and three weeks after surgery she was swimming and cycling. In contrast Denise was unable to leave her bed for fourteen days after her hysterectomy. She convalesced slowly at home and finally returned to work thirteen weeks after surgery. The variation in the physical recovery of Rosa and Denise demonstrates why it is difficult for a surgeon to provide a fixed schedule for post-operative recovery.

To do so might put the brakes on the recovery of some women and unduly tax the capabilities of others.

Women recover from hysterectomy at different rates for many reasons. These include the nature and severity of the problem for which the operation was carried out, the type of operation performed and the extent to which it interfered with various organs of the body, the skill of the surgeon, the general physical and psychological health of the woman pre-operatively and the effect of anaesthetic agents on her.

Pain relief

An important guiding principle to remember is that when the wound is healed physical activity can do no harm; it can actually play an important part in the healing process. Pain is a good guide to wound healing and will usually indicate what is feasible. If you want to walk, try it. If it causes pain, take a rest. When you can walk easily, try a new activity requiring a little more physical exertion. While pain relief after surgery makes it more difficult to judge when the wound has healed, it has other important benefits. **Jan was extremely reluctant to accept pain relief after her hysterectomy and wanted to do without painkillers if at all possible. The only problem with this approach was that it caused Jan to restrict her movements to minimise the pain. This resulted in the formation of a blood clot that settled in her leg. She was persuaded that pain relief would enable her to move about and this seemed to short-circuit further clot problems.**

Thrombosis

Thrombosis, the formation of blood clots within a blood vessel, is one of the most dangerous complications of any type of surgery. The pelvis or leg are the most common sites of thrombosis after major abdominal surgery. If the thrombosis is swept along by the bloodstream, it can lodge in the lungs blocking the circulation and depriving the body of oxygen. Measures which reduce the risk of thrombosis are described in chapter 7.

Lung complications

Lung complications such as pneumonia or lung collapse occur very rarely after a hysterectomy. If you have a bad cold in the days before you are due for your operation, let your doctor know so that a new time can be made. It is also important to stop smoking at least one week before surgery.

Bowel function

Restoring normal function to the body is the crux of recuperation. Bowel function is less active than usual for a day or so after hysterectomy due to the effects of the anaesthetic and the handling of internal organs during surgery. For this reason, food is vetoed and fluids are restricted for anything up to twenty-four hours after surgery. In order to provide adequate nourishment during this time an intravenous drip is connected to a vein in the arm. Once bowel activity starts — and this is helped by getting up and moving around — fluid intake can be increased and light meals started. Many women experience distress at this time due to large amounts of 'wind' and colicky pain which usually last for one to three days. Strategies to overcome these side-effects include pain relief which may come in tablet form or, in severe cases, injections. Some pain killers, such as codeine, are best avoided because they can cause constipation. Charcoal tablets, which absorb gas in the bowel, can alleviate this problem very effectively. A mild laxative is often found helpful or, if difficulty persists, a suppository. Strong laxatives and enemas may

be used when there is a prolonged delay in bowel emptying, particularly if this is associated with colic. It is not
unusual for bowel function to take several months to
return to normal after hysterectomy.

On rare occasions, the bowel may be paralysed for several days after surgery. Eating will stretch the paralysed
bowel and cause further delays in recovery of bowel function. So an intravenous drip is needed to supply nutritional needs in the meantime. Another rare occurrence is
bowel blockage caused by the formation of adhesions
during the operation. The blockage may resolve if the
bowel is rested, but if not, further surgery is required.
Although this is an unusual and unpleasant complication, the outcome is generally quite satisfactory.

Bladder function

Bladder function may also be affected following hysterectomy due to bruising of the bladder or damage to
the nerves and blood vessels that connect it to other
organs. The resulting difficulty in emptying the bladder
may be overcome by inserting a catheter (tube) into
the bladder. In some women the bladder is rested for
several days and the catheter drains urine continuously
into a closed bag beside the bed. When the catheter is
removed the bladder sometimes goes 'on strike' and is
difficult to empty. A physiotherapist can help ease any
discomfort by encouraging full relaxation of the pelvic
floor muscles and applying gentle diaphragm pressure
from above. Because of bruising, damage to nerves or
changes in anatomy following hysterectomy, bladder
function may not return to normal until one or two
months after surgery. It is extremely important to
practise pelvic floor and abdominal exercises (see chapter 6) once healing is complete. Not only do they help

with bladder control, they also enhance muscular support for the newly positioned organs.

A bladder infection may complicate matters, causing a feeling of scalding when urine is passed, a feeling of wanting to pass urine frequently or pain. The doctor will send a specimen of urine for laboratory examination and will prescribe an appropriate antibiotic to clear the bladder of any infection that is found.

Vaginal discharge

A yellow and unpleasant smelling vaginal discharge can occur if the wound at the top of the vagina (produced during an abdominal or laparoscopically assisted hysterectomy) becomes infected. This wound generally takes longer to heal than an abdominal scar and the moisture of the vagina can encourage bacterial growth. It is quite normal to have a red- or brown-staining discharge for anything from two to eight weeks after a hysterectomy. But if it becomes smelly and yellow, or persists beyond this time, it should be checked by a doctor. Sometimes a small amount of flesh forms along the edge of the wound and this can be removed painlessly by diathermy.

Scarring

The top of the vagina may be narrowed or shortened as a result of the hysterectomy and any scar in that area may take as long as three months to lose its tenderness and become flexible. Occasionally the hysterectomy itself leads to a prolapse of the bladder, rectum or vagina (see chapter 2). Further surgery is then needed to reposition and anchor the organs so that they do not collapse downwards. Resumption of sexual intercourse and issues concerning sexuality after a hysterectomy are discussed in chapter 6.

Various problems can occur with an abdominal scar, especially if a woman has previously had several abdominal operations (for example, Caesarean sections). The scar may be itchy or sore and the woman may think it looks unsightly. Some physiotherapists use ultrasound to soften the scar tissue and ease the soreness. The sound waves that are generated during ultrasound have a mechanical shaking effect which stimulates blood flow and cell activity in the hardened areas. Sometimes it is possible to reposition the scar or combine a number of scars during further surgery. Bruising and swelling at the site of an incision may also pose problems. The area may be drained or left to resolve itself, a process that can take several months.

Hormonal effects and other considerations

Emotional highs and lows are common after hysterectomy with many women experiencing tearfulness and irritability. One explanation is the stress of the surgery and the effect of the anaesthetic. In addition, the removal of the ovaries, or their inadvertent damage, will quickly lead to changes in sex hormone levels and, with this, mood fluctuations.

Hot flushes, night sweats and associated sleeplessness may follow close on the heels of a hysterectomy, particularly if the ovaries have been removed. These effects are blamed on rapid changes in the levels of oestrogen, progesterone and other sex hormones circulating in the bloodstream. The symptoms diminish over the space of months or years but they can play havoc with the lives of women and their loved ones until then. Hormone therapy is often regarded as a simple solution to these problems and in some women this appears to be the case. Others, however, cannot tolerate hormone therapy or they may be concerned about possible long-term effects, for example the increased risk of developing breast cancer with prolonged (more than five years) use of hormone therapy.

On returning home, some women expect to resume everyday activities without missing a beat. Unfortunately, pain or other problems may prevent this and partners, children and relatives should be on call to lend a hand. If this sort of help is not available, it may be possible to arrange for assistance from the local council, a nursing service or another organisation. The decision about when to resume driving is important as lives can hinge on it. Emergency braking requires quick reflexes and leg strength. By the time women are able to climb stairs quickly and do the garden, they are usually fit enough to drive.

Time spent in hospital and recovering

Most women having an abdominal hysterectomy will spend about seven to ten days in hospital, with a somewhat shorter stay (one to four days) if they have a laparoscopically assisted hysterectomy. Two out of three women having an abdominal hysterectomy resume pre-hysterectomy activities in about three months, with the remainder needing longer, perhaps up to a year.

Vaginal hysterectomy avoids the pelvic incision of abdominal hysterectomy and consequently postoperative pain may be reduced. The hospital stay (about seven days) and recovery period (four to six weeks) also tend to be shorter. Laparoscopically assisted hysterectomy requires an even shorter hospital stay (usually less than four days) and usually ensures a more rapid return to full function.

Financial considerations

The health care costs of abdominal, vaginal and laparoscopically assisted hysterectomies are comparable. However the reduced recovery time of the latter approach promises considerable benefits to women, their families and employers.

An economic evaluation that compared the costs of abdominal hysterectomy and endometrial resection in England for the four months up to and including surgery, found total costs for the former were nearly twice that of the latter.[10] The authors suggested, however, this was not the end of the story:

> Given the fact that a subgroup of women requires re-treatment due to resection failure and that this study considers a relatively short period of follow-up, the long-term costs and benefits of endometrial resection need to be evaluated before widespread diffusion is justified.

The all-up cost of an abdominal hysterectomy in Australia in 1993 was about $5000, and for a vaginal hysterectomy it was considerably less at $3550. The cost of a laparoscopically assisted hysterectomy was about $5700, of which almost $1200 was for disposable instruments. Women who do not have private health insurance and whose hysterectomy is carried out in a public hospital can expect to pay nothing. Women with private health insurance can expect to pay $500 or more, regardless of whether they attend a public or private hospital. Their payment will depend on their level of insurance and the fees charged by their surgeon and anaesthetist. Uninsured patients having a hysterectomy in a private hospital face payments of $2500 to $3000.

five

Making the treatment decision

Each year hundreds of thousands of women worldwide have their uterus surgically removed, many find the experience a landmark event. Some feel very positively about it, others have mixed feelings, and some experience intense regret. Deciding whether or not to have a hysterectomy and which type is most suitable can be difficult, especially when the views of trusted advisers are in conflict. **In the case of Lisa, aged forty-two, friends, relatives, her partner and doctor held strong but differing opinions about the merits and drawbacks of the procedure. Some were enthusiastic about it, others thought there were other options, such as endometrial resection, that Lisa should investigate before agreeing to the removal of her uterus. Still others were adamant that hysterectomy was only to be considered in the most exceptional circumstances which, they assured Lisa, hers were not. She felt confused, a feeling made worse by criticism from her doctor that she was talking to too many people who lacked information about risks, success rates and alternatives. Lisa was not at all sure that facts and figures about risks, benefits and other options were the** only considerations that were valid. She wondered, for example, whether various social stresses in her life were affecting the way she felt about her symptoms.

The distress of women who, like Lisa, are in the invidious position of having to decide whether to have a hysterectomy or find other ways of resolving their problems is evident. Even women who have an intimate acquaintance with the anatomy of the female pelvis can find the situation daunting. For example, when Sydney gynaecologist Caroline de Costa was contemplating a hysterectomy in 1992, she was nagged by fears right up to her arrival in the operating theatre.

The story told by de Costa, one of the few gynaecologists in Australia ever to have had a hysterectomy, reflects the anguish and ambivalence of many women contemplating the procedure.[1] One of her fears was that she would feel enormous regret for the loss of her uterus and for her inability to bear any further children. She told herself this was ridiculous — at forty-five years of age and with seven children spaced over twenty-four years, why not put an end to the increasingly long, heavy and painful periods she was experiencing more and more often? De Costa also had a prolapsed uterus, had postponed her decision for several years and felt it was irrational to delay having the operation any longer. Another lingering concern was how she would actually feel, within her abdomen and pelvis, once her uterus was removed. 'Perhaps there was something my patients hadn't told me,' she thought. 'Perhaps I will feel a kind of black hole between my bladder and bowel.'

The experience of contemplating a hysterectomy over a long time, then going ahead with it, brought home to de Costa the emotional turmoil that many women in the same situation go through. It resulted in a change in the way in which she conducted her consultations. 'I am certainly spending more time now in discussion with patients in an attempt to allay these fears,' she said after making a full recovery and returning to her practice.

The decision-making process

Women consider having a hysterectomy for reasons such as chronic abdominal pain and excessive bleeding, and because of a doctor's recommendation. Non-medical reasons may also influence the advice of medical practitioners, and of a woman's family and friends. According to recent Australian and US studies, a doctor's advice about hysterectomy may have more influence on a woman's decision about surgery than her understanding of the reason(s) for the operation, its probable after-effects, or the alternatives available. Presumably, a doctor's recommendation for a non-surgical approach may be equally persuasive.

Dorothy's 'decision' to have a hysterectomy followed her admission to hospital to have bladder repair surgery. The night before the operation her doctor visited her and, as he was leaving, said casually, 'We might as well take your womb out while we're in there, because you don't have any need for it now.' When asked how she felt about this, Dorothy said she accepted it without question because she believed her doctor knew what was best.

There is no doubt that some women prefer to leave decisions about their health care entirely to their doctors, even to the extent of preferring the doctor to decide whether or not they should have major surgery. But it is becoming increasingly common for doctors and women to work together, exchanging information and ideas and, in the end, coming to a mutual agreement about the best course of action.

Psychologists have identified five basic patterns of behaviour used by individuals when faced with choices about things like health investigations and treatments.

- Complacently continuing whatever has been familiar until then, which may involve discounting new and relevant information.
- Uncritically adopting whichever new course of action is most strongly recommended or is considered to be 'the fashion'.
- Escaping the conflict by delaying decision making, shifting the responsibility to someone else, or making wishful excuses to bolster a particular alternative, meanwhile refusing to consider pertinent information.
- Searching frantically for a way out of the dilemma and impulsively seizing upon a hasty solution that seems to promise immediate relief. This type of decision making means that the full range of consequences of a particular choice are never considered.
- Searching painstakingly for relevant information, thinking carefully about it in as unbiased a way as possible, and weighing the alternatives carefully before making a choice.

Although the first two patterns may save time, effort and emotional turmoil, they often lead to decision making that is less than ideal and has unfortunate consequences. The third and fourth patterns likewise tend to be associated with undesirable results. The fifth pattern, termed the 'vigilant approach', usually leads to high-quality decision making. Its major features include identifying the feasible options; sorting out personal values, objectives, barriers to particular actions and incentives to others; assessing the consequences of a particular choice; planning how best to put the decision into effect; and anticipating what will happen as a result of that decision.

Today, many women are participating actively and responsibly in making decisions about their health and are having a major say about investigations and treatments. Your consent should always be sought before a procedure is carried out, except in the most unusual of circumstances, such as an emergency during major surgery when your life would be threatened if a particular action was not taken. In addition, your consent should always be sought for participation in medical research. Remember also that it is your right to withdraw from treatment by a particular practitioner at any time.

For most women, a decision for or against a hysterectomy involves the following considerations:

- an assessment of the impact of the existing medical condition and its symptoms on quality of life
- a comparison of physical risks and effectiveness of various forms of treatment
- a personal assessment of the importance of the uterus and of emotional reactions to the current situation and to removal of the uterus
- careful consideration of any relevant social and cultural factors
- the views of a doctor or doctors, a partner and close friends
- an assessment of the skill and care of medical personnel available to you.

Non-medical reasons for hysterectomy

The continuing debate about whether hysterectomy is overused is an issue of great importance for the many women who will ask themselves at some time in their lives, 'Is a hysterectomy really necessary for me?' The debate has been fuelled by findings of large variations in rates of hysterectomy between and within countries for no apparent reason. The United States has the highest rate, followed by Canada, New Zealand, Australia, Holland, England, Wales, Scotland, Sweden and Japan. The disparities are large, with at least three women in the US having hysterectomies for every one in Scotland, and Coloured women traditionally having twice as many as White women.

Various suggestions have been made to account for these differences in hysterectomy rates. It is possible that there are specific inherited tendencies for the development of certain gynaecological diseases in different countries and ethnic groups. Equally, the explanation may lie in environmental factors or lifestyle habits, for example nutrition, physical activity levels, or even methods of sanitary protection or contraception. Perhaps women in some countries are more assertive in taking control of their lives and bodies; or maybe cultural differences in perceptions of the uterus are important — some cultures viewing it as essential to womanhood, others regarding it as an optional extra once the desired family size is reached. Other plausible explanations for variations in rates of hysterectomy are that views about what constitutes a 'normal' bleeding pattern differ from country to country as does the acceptability of menstrual disturbances within intimate relationships and the paid workforce. Yet other reasons suggested for the large variations in rates of hysterectomy include different opinions about its acceptability as a sterilisation procedure, particularly among couples for whom religious beliefs preclude other forms of family planning.

Fashions in gynaecology may also be influential, resulting in certain symptoms being regarded as signs of 'disease' in one country or era but not in another. For example, in the late nineteenth century heavy bleeding in middle-aged women was said to be responsible for heart flutters, delusions and nervousness. Unable to replace the blood, doctors resorted to all kinds of techniques to stop the bleeding. These included hysterectomy and radiological methods of inducing menopause such as bombarding the ovaries with X-rays or placing radium rods in the vagina. A contemporary example of changing medical definitions of illness is the recent claim that menopause constitutes a 'disease' and that the cure is to prescribe hormone therapy for all women. This may have implications for hysterectomy rates because, as noted by the US Congress Office of Technology Assessment, women receiving hormone therapy are more likely to undergo hysterectomy, possibly because bleeding is a common side-effect of its use.[2]

It has also been claimed that some health systems encourage high rates of hysterectomy through methods of health financing that encourage swift surgical 'solutions' rather than more prolonged treatments; the expectations of surgeons that hysterectomy should be part of their professional work and source of income; the availability of hospital beds; and the extent to which doctors get paid for the number of operations they perform.[3]

Yet another explanation for high hysterectomy rates is that women who consent to the operation are not informed of, or lack the resources to find out about, non-surgical options for treating their problems. Most studies that have examined the characteristics of women who have hysterectomies are in agreement on one point at least — the fewer the years of high school or college education, the more likely a woman is to have a hysterectomy.[4] Complementing this finding, a recent study in the US State of Maine has found that better-educated women are more likely to have non-surgical treatments for fibroids, abnormal bleeding or chronic pelvic pain, all common reasons for hysterectomies.[5] In view of the consistent link between lower education levels and hysterectomy, it is difficult to explain the seemingly contradictory finding that the wives of medical practitioners have more hysterectomies proportionately than other well-educated groups in the US.[6]

Another interesting finding to come out of the Maine study is that women who agree to hysterectomies have symptoms that are both more severe and more incapacitating than women who seek relief through non-surgical approaches.[7] They often endure debilitating symptoms for several years before deciding on hysterectomy. Other studies have revealed that women having the surgery are more likely than average to be overweight, to have diabetes or to have high blood pressure.[8] With some notable exceptions, such as US doctors' wives, hysterectomy, poor health and low education levels seem to go hand in hand. Researchers studying the phenomenon of hysterectomy rate variations agree that no simple explanation can account for these differences.

Trends in hysterectomy

More than 25 000 Australian women had hysterectomies in 1975 and at that rate it was estimated that at least four out of every ten would have this form of surgery by the time they turned sixty-five.[9] Twenty years later, with an ageing population that includes a high proportion of older women, it is estimated that 30 000 hysterectomies are performed in Australia annually.[10]

Current evidence suggests that 20–30% of Australian women will have a hysterectomy during their lifetime, usually between their mid-thirties and mid-fifties.[11] About three-quarters of these are performed before women go through a natural menopause, that is, before their menstrual periods stop of their own accord. The Melbourne Women's Midlife Health Project is documenting the situation in 2000 randomly selected Melbourne women aged from forty-five to fifty-five. The Project, undertaken by the Key Centre for Women's Health in Society at the University of Melbourne, has found a 22% rate of hysterectomy among the women, and a peak age for the operation of just over forty years.[12]

Another study, conducted by the Australian Institute of Health and Welfare, suggests that one explanation for an apparent downward trend in hysterectomy rates in Australia is the rapid introduction of the surgical procedures known as endometrial resection and ablation, described in detail in chapter 3.[13] This study has found that approximately 4000 Medicare benefit payments were made for endometrial resection in 1991–92, and in the same period the rate of hysterectomy (for heavy, uncontrolled bleeding) in public hospitals in Australia declined by one-third. Although the effects of endometrial resection on bleeding patterns are still being evaluated and the technique itself is still undergoing development, it appears to offer a credible alternative to hysterectomy for some women. Equally, it is fairly certain that hysterectomy will never be eliminated completely. For the several thousand women in Australia each year who are diagnosed as having cancer of the cervix or of the endometrium, survival itself may rely on a hysterectomy.

Recently, there has been a surge of interest in new treatment alternatives to hysterectomy, some of which are surgical, while others are psychological, medical and lifestyle-oriented. At the same time as we applaud the effort that is going into developing new or revamped treatment approaches, we believe that significant information gaps remain about their long-term safety and effectiveness. Research needs to continue and women must be informed of the current gaps in medical knowledge when making treatment decisions.

What to look for in a practitioner

If frank discussions with your medical adviser are important to you, then your doctor needs to be a person with whom you can comfortably discuss all relevant issues and who takes the time and effort to answer your questions. Sometimes the information a practitioner provides does not stick the first time and, as Toni found, a doctor's patience and understanding are important. 'I felt embarrassed above all else,' Toni recalled. 'I had seen my gynaecologist and we talked about the pros and cons of a hysterectomy. I asked a lot of questions, but when I came home and tried to remember his answers, there was so much I had forgotten. Maybe it was because I was feeling depressed or perhaps I wasn't really ready to consider that sort of surgery. When I went back and asked many of the same questions all over again, he put me at ease by reassuring me that it was not at all unusual and quite important to cover the same ground several times.' You should not hesitate to ask for another appointment if the consultation ends before questions or issues are resolved to your satisfaction. Alternatively, a gynaecologist will often suggest a second or third appointment when the possibility of a hysterectomy is being considered.

An essential quality in any health practitioner is good communication skills. He or she should listen carefully to what you have to say and give you a clear explanation of the possible or likely nature of your illness or disease. Together you should discuss the proposed approach to tests, diagnosis and treatment, including what the proposed approach entails; the expected benefits, common side-effects and risks; whether the intervention is conventional or experimental; and who will undertake it. Your practitioner should raise with you, or you should ask about, other options for investigation, diagnosis and treatment. Another important attribute of a practitioner is the ability to convey information in an effective yet sensitive manner and to recognise what you have gone through already and may yet go through. A practitioner who is unable to put him- or herself in your shoes is less likely to understand your preferences or needs. If there are language difficulties between you and your practitioner, encourage the doctor to arrange for an interpreter to be present or, if this is not possible, bring someone with you who can translate.

Once a diagnosis has been arrived at, you should be informed of any uncertainties about that, or about the outcome of any treatment proposed. You need to be sure that the outcome expected from the treatment is compatible with what you want from treatment. For example, if you still desire children and you do not have a life-threatening cancer, a hysterectomy is not a sensible first option for you. The doctor may want to discuss the likely consequences if you do not choose to have a proposed treatment. The expected time to recovery and financial costs are matters that you may also need to discuss. In addition, it is particularly important that you satisfy yourself that the doctor is experienced and skilful in the job to be done, and that any significant risk of long-term physical, emotional, social, sexual or other outcome is known to you.

The issue of what constitutes a 'significant risk' received lengthy consideration during a recent Australian High Court decision (*Rogers v. Whitaker* [1992]). The case concerned a woman who was blinded by the treatment she received, a less than one in 1000 chance in her particular case. The presiding judge defined the risks to be discussed by a doctor with his or her patient as those which, in the circumstances of the particular case, a reasonable person in the patient's position would be likely to attach significance to if warned of the risk.

In practice, some doctors seem to think they should have control over what is discussed. A 1993 study of over 1000 doctors, conducted for Australian federal health authorities, found that 84% considered there were circumstances in which they would be justified in withholding information.[14] Some of the reasons given seem questionable at best. About a third of the doctors said they would consider withholding information if they thought a patient might refuse treatment, while between a third and a half would consider withholding information if they regarded the patient as a poor decision-maker. Only half of the doctors surveyed said they always discussed the risk of death or serious disability where it occurred at least as often as once in every 100 cases. For lower risks of death or disability (one in 1000 was specified) less than a quarter of the doctors said that they always discussed these with patients. On a more hopeful note, another Australian study of doctors found that the most significant changes to medical practice over a recent five year period were 'taking more time to explain risks' and 'spending more time on patient record keeping'.[15]

Before making decisions about treatment, it is a help if your doctor draws a picture of the suggested treatment approach if this is possible (and it certainly is where surgery is involved), and gives you written materials to take home and think about. If you are unsure, ask more questions. If you are still undecided, ask for time to make up your mind. Don't be hurried. Except in the case of a diagnosed cancer, time is on your side.

If you need to go to a clinic or a hospital for treatment, the practitioner should provide you with clear information about any pre-treatment requirements (such as stopping the Pill a month before major surgery, stopping smoking at least a week beforehand, and refraining from food and drink from the night before a general anaesthetic). You should also be given details of your continuing health care, for example post-treatment check-ups, once you are discharged from a clinic or hospital.

Overseas studies and case study research suggest that most formal complaints issued by patients about their doctors arise from situations where there has been a failure of communication. If things do not go to plan, your practitioner should carefully and fully explain what went wrong and should deal with you openly and fairly.

Finding a health practitioner

Consumer organisations usually recommend that the first step to finding a health practitioner who suits your needs is a recommendation from someone whose judgement you trust. Your general practitioner may know of a gynaecologist who has expertise in treating your condition; although general practitioners sometimes ask patients if they know of anyone suitable. In this case, you might like to put forward the name of a gynaecologist who has been recommended to you by other women in your family or by your friends. If you have any doubts about whether the specialist recommended has suitable experience, you can check whether he or she belongs to the relevant professional association, such as the national College of Obstetricians and Gynaecologists, and then ring that association and check that his or her training and qualifications are adequate.

The consumer guide *Choice* advises patients choosing a practitioner in alternative medicine to check if the relevant professional association has a code of ethics, disciplinary procedures for practitioners who break the code, and a complaints procedure for dissatisfied clients. 'These factors aren't a guarantee', *Choice* says, 'but indicate the organisation is serious about maintaining high professional standards.'[16]

It does not bode well if you feel inhibited, rushed or unsettled with a particular practitioner or if he or she does not treat you with respect, dignity and consideration for your privacy. This is your cue to look elsewhere for help. Equally, it is reasonable to bypass any practitioner who suggests a treatment that seems extreme or very expensive, who speaks in incomprehensible jargon or who recommends a single treatment for all women. Sometimes a practitioner will recommend a particular treatment not because it is particularly well suited to your needs but because he or she is able to give that treatment or it is available nearby. Questioning your practitioner about why one particular treatment is preferable to others can be revealing.

Getting a second opinion

If you are uncertain about whether to have a particular treatment, you should take the time to discuss the issues with your general practitioner and perhaps a second specialist. Either your general practitioner or the first specialist may refer you to a second specialist. If the first specialist refers you to another specialist for a second opinion, it is a good idea to ask the referring specialist if he or she still wishes to perform a procedure recommended by the second specialist.

A second opinion is worthwhile because doctors often disagree on the appropriateness of major surgery like hysterectomy in a given situation. You may find after consulting the second doctor that you have two completely different views about the course of action you should follow. In this case, you may find your general practitioner can help you decide between the two opinions by encouraging you to examine carefully your own needs and situation. If you decide to accept a treatment approach suggested by a second specialist, you can choose treatment from the specialist you prefer. The second specialist should notify both your general practitioner and the first specialist of his or her findings and recommendations.

Suggested questions for your practitioner

If you are considering any sort of investigation or treatment, Australia's National Health and Medical Research Council recommends that you ask your practitioner the following sorts of questions:

- What is the possible or likely nature of my illness or disease?
- What is your proposed approach to investigation, diagnosis and treatment?
  — what does this approach entail?
  — what are its expected benefits?

— what are the common side-effects and risks of the intervention proposed?
— is the intervention a standard procedure or is it experimental?
— who will carry out the intervention? How much of that particular procedure has that person performed? And with what results, including rates of complications in her/his series of patients. (If he/she doesn't know, this may indicate a reluctance to self-monitor and may be a bad sign.)

- What are the other options for investigation, diagnosis and treatment?
- How certain is the diagnosis?
- How certain is the treatment outcome?
- What is likely to happen if the proposed investigation or treatment does not occur, or if no procedure or treatment is undertaken?
- What significant long-term effects may be associated with particular investigations or treatments?
- How much time is involved in conducting particular investigations or treatments, and in recovering from them?
- What costs are involved, including costs payable after receiving Medicare and health-insurance rebates?

If you find it difficult to ask these sorts of questions, take someone along with you who can.

The decision-making checklist

Deciding between the different sorts of treatment options described in this book will involve weighing up the positives and negatives as you see them. The simple checklist that follows may be of use to you in this decision-making process. It may help to crystallise your thinking or it may suggest gaps in information that need to be filled before you can make a firm decision.

Step 1

Write the name of the treatment that has been suggested to you in the space provided.

Step 2

Following are two lists of possible outcomes. They have been grouped together as possible reasons in favour of a proposed treatment (pro) and against a proposed treatment (con). Space has been left for any additional pros and cons that you may need to include. Read through the lists and place a tick alongside any pro or con that is relevant to you. Leave a blank if that consideration has no importance one way or the other. If you do not have enough information to tick a line or leave it blank, place a question mark next to it to remind you to seek more information on it.

Step 3

Identify the most important pro and the most important con for you (highlighting or underlining them with a coloured pen may be helpful) and compare their importance.

Step 4

Select the next most important pro and con (using a different coloured pen), and then the next most important pair, and so on.

By continuing this process, it should be possible to decide whether the pros clearly outweigh the cons or

The suggested treatment is ....

Possible pro outcomes
* No more bleeding
* Relief from other symptoms (e.g. pain)
* Further gynaecological operations unlikely
* Pregnancy no longer possible
* Pap smears not needed
* Endometrial cancer risk eliminated
* Improvement in sexual satisfaction for self or partner
* Maintenance of intact reproductive system
* Agrees with opinion of important others
* Acceptable financial cost

....
....

Possible con outcomes
* Failure of symptom relief
* Ongoing medical consultations or investigations needed
* Surgery and anaesthetic required
* Drug therapy needed
* Pregnancy no longer possible
* Immediate risks and complications of treatment
* Disagrees with opinion of important others
* May reduce sexual satisfaction for self or partner
* Need for home help during recovery
* Financial cost of procedure (including time off work if applicable)
* Anticipated time of recuperation
* Possibility of earlier menopause
* Possible long-term increased risk of osteoporosis, heart disease or cancer

....
....

Issues on which I need more information

....
....

The balance between the pros and cons as I see it

....
....

vice-versa, or whether they are relatively even. If there is a definite loading one way or the other, you will be more certain of the reasons for accepting or rejecting a particular treatment. On the other hand, you may be alerted to questions that you need to have answered before you can make a decision.

You will notice that identical or similar possible outcomes appear in both the pro and con lists from time to time. This helps make the point that, for example, 'Pregnancy no longer possible' is a pro for some women at a particular age and stage of life and a con for other women in different circumstances.

A final word

To give yourself the best chance of 'getting it right':
- communicate your problems and needs clearly and as often as necessary
- make use of all the services available
- be realistic — treatment miracles don't exist and no treatment is perfect
- develop a web of support for yourself
- remember what you can do, rather than focusing on what you can't.

six

Issues for women and their sexual partners

One of the questions many women ask about hysterectomy is the effect of the surgery on their sexuality, sexual interest, satisfaction and response. Because these areas of a woman's life are usually shared, sexual partners also have an interest in the answers. This chapter presents information on what is known of the positive and negative effects of hysterectomy on sexuality and sexual function, and explores measures to improve the situation should problems arise. Information, where available, is included about the impact on sexuality and sexual function of various other types of gynaecological surgery such as the removal of fibroids, and of drug treatments such as those which reduce bleeding.

It is important to note at the outset that studies of sexual behaviour are a relatively recent phenomenon in human history, one reason being that many people have reservations about studying something they regard as intrinsically private. The upshot is that much of the information we have on sexual behaviour comes from groups of volunteers who may not be representative of the population in general. It is important to remember this in drawing conclusions from such studies.

The studies of Alfred Kinsey and his associates in the 1940s and 1950s were more wide-ranging than most studies before or since. His team asked more than 5900 White American women and 5300 White American men about their sexual practices and found, among other things, that women and men reported a decline in sex drive as they got older. Sexual activity in old age was related to sexual activity earlier in life, with those having an active sex life in old age more likely to have been sexually active during their youth and middle years.

Some people place enormous store on maintaining an active sex life into old age, while for others it is neither here nor there. Views on this are diverse, and we do not wish to suggest that sex is a requirement for a happy and satisfying life. People who have no desire for, or interest in, sex or who have deliberately chosen a lifestyle in which sexual activities play little or no part, have every right to their decision. The obverse is also true. Older people who enjoy sex, or who want to enjoy it in a mutually satisfying relationship, should be given information to help them achieve this.

Effect of hysterectomy on sexuality and sexual function

For most women, hysterectomy does not adversely affect sexuality. In studies of the effects of the operation on sexual interest and response, a minority of women — between 7 and 20% depending on the study — report some decrease in sexual function after hysterectomy. About the same proportion report an improvement, and more than half report no change. When partners of women who have had the operation are asked about its impact on sexuality, many have no comment, over a third say they are happy their partners had the operation for reasons such as removal of the fear of an unwanted pregnancy. A small minority express dissatisfaction saying things like the vagina is 'too tight' or 'too dry'.

Although the overwhelming consensus from recent studies that have followed women through the experience of hysterectomy is of a clear reduction in the disabling symptoms that lead to surgery, many women continue to have concerns about the effects of hysterectomy on sexuality and sexual function. The picture is complex because at around the age when most women have a hysterectomy they may also be starting or passing through menopause. The changes associated with this transition may themselves have an impact on sexuality and sexual function and these may be incorrectly blamed on the hysterectomy.

Doctors have been aware of sexual difficulties in a minority of women who have had a hysterectomy and have sometimes attributed it to post-surgical depression or concerns about self-image. These conclusions have been questioned in recent years, with an increasing number of medical practitioners and sex therapists suggesting that the procedure itself contributes to post-surgical difficulties in some women. Our ignorance of the role of the uterus and cervix in sexual response may be partly responsible for the occurrence of these difficulties.

A generation ago, it was believed that a woman's major sexual response was centred in her clitoris and vagina. Recent research suggests, however, that for some women there are sexual sensations associated with the uterus itself. In the process of performing a hysterectomy, major arteries, veins and nerves that flow to and from the uterus are inevitably cut. It is possible that this interference may play a role in the sexual dysfunction reported by some women after hysterectomy. For some men, too, sexual satisfaction and response may be influenced by the presence of the cervix, against which the penis taps during intercourse.

There are several main ways in which hysterectomy can change sexual response. These changes may be either positive or negative.

- Removal of the fear of pregnancy may allow women and their partners to engage in sex with fewer inhibitions.
- Reduction or elimination of heavy and prolonged menstrual bleeding may enhance the experience of orgasm and intercourse.
- This same positive outcome may occur as a result of removing adhesions, fibroids and other causes of chronic pelvic pain when the uterus is taken.
- Alteration of the size and shape of the vagina during the surgery may make the sensations associated with sex more or less pleasurable for one or both partners.
- Removal of the main part of the uterus may eliminate pleasurable sensations associated with its contraction and movement. These sensations may occur during sexual foreplay, for example when the clitoris, breasts, vulva and vagina are touched, as well as during intercourse.
- Removal of the cervix may reduce sexual satisfaction. This is because of the pleasure that a woman and her partner may derive from the tapping of the penis on the cervix during intercourse.
- Creation of new scar tissue in the pelvis or vagina as a result of a hysterectomy may cause intercourse to become more painful.
- Changes in hormone production, particularly marked if the ovaries are removed at the time of the hysterec-

tomy, may lead to intercourse becoming less pleasurable. These hormone changes — which tend to be more acute than when menopause occurs without surgical intervention — may result in several ill-effects. Decreased oestrogen levels may be associated with a general drying and thinning of the vagina. This may in turn result in painful intercourse, and severe night sweats and insomnia leading to feelings of fatigue. A decreased output of androgen hormones, including testosterone, by the ovaries may also reduce sexual interest (libido) in women.

- Psychological effects on either partner, related to feelings of loss of the uterus, may lead to decreased pleasure in intercourse. This is more likely to occur if intercourse has been valued mainly for the children that may result from it.

The preceding discussion has assumed heterosexual sexual behaviour. However, not everyone is primarily attracted to members of the opposite sex; some people, both males and females, are aroused by and form homosexual relationships with members of their own sex. Research on the effects of hysterectomy on the sexual relationships of lesbian women is extremely limited and deserves more attention.

Another area in which knowledge is limited is the previously mentioned role of the uterus in sexual response. As indicated in chapter 4, there is growing evidence that the uterus is involved in orgasm, at least in a proportion of women. Direct stimulation of the cervix during sexual intercourse also seems to have a role in the sexual response of some women and men.

More information exists about the effects of changes in hormone production after hysterectomy. Even when the ovaries are retained, oestrogen levels seem to be affected by hysterectomy in some women. About a quarter of women whose ovaries remain after hysterectomy experience early loss of ovarian function (on average four to five years earlier than in comparable women who have not had a hysterectomy) which can lead to vaginal dryness and hot flushes. In a bid to prevent or overcome these problems, many women with indications of low oestrogen levels are prescribed oestrogen therapy after a hysterectomy whether or not their ovaries have been removed.

A woman's attitudes — and those of her partner — can be an extremely important influence on sexual relations after hysterectomy. In the aftermath of her hysterectomy, Kay was already questioning her femininity and attractiveness. She had regarded her main role in life as childbearing and suddenly, without the ability to do this, her life lost meaning. But her agitation grew when Kevin failed to respond to her attempts to arouse him sexually. She worried that she was now less attractive to him and new tensions entered their relationship. This unfortunate chain of events continued until the couple sat down and communicated their feelings and fears; Kevin explaining that he was worried about causing Kay pain when they made love, Kay coming to grips with the reasons why Kevin and others valued her.

In the case of Vin, talking did not help a great deal. He thought his wife Mary was less of a woman after undergoing hysterectomy but found it difficult to say exactly why. He understood that Mary had tried many other approaches to resolving her medical problems without success, and that something had to be done to relieve her pain and bleeding. In cases such as this, it can be helpful if a spouse or partner is involved in the decision-making process, thus providing opportunities to discuss any concerns with the doctor. It may also alert women to the need for a concerted effort on all sides to overcome unforeseen barriers to re-establishing a satisfactory sexual relationship.

Effect of other treatments on sexuality and sexual function

Any major gynaecological surgery, such as an open myomectomy which entails a large incision and a general anaesthetic, will put sex off the agenda for at least six to eight weeks. This does not mean you cannot enjoy each other in intimate ways. The opportunity to give pleasure to each other through massage can help the recovery process. It can also help the sexual relationship in the longer term by allowing partners to communicate their sexual needs to each other and learn about each other's sexual responses before sexual intercourse resumes.

One type of activity that most couples find enjoyable, starts with partners giving each other a general body massage. Hand cream or body oil, and an atmosphere that is warm and relaxed, will add to the experience. As the massage occurs, the partner who is being stroked and rubbed describes his or her feelings and desires. In this way each partner learns how the other likes to be stimulated and caressed and unexplored areas of communication and fantasy may be unearthed. The activity may continue to climax.

After a hysterectomy, hysteroscopy, laparoscopy, endometrial ablation or endometrial resection, the desire to give and receive love remains. Most people want to continue with intimacy — the challenge is to be flexible enough to manage this when some of the old ways of being intimate are on hold. Giving and gaining pleasure may be achieved by caressing, cuddling and enjoying each other's company. The use of a hand-held vibrator on many parts of the body can arouse sensations in areas we do not usually think of as pleasure zones, such as the soles of the feet, the face and the lips. Intercourse can be resumed when bleeding or discharge has stopped and the pelvis feels normal. Depending on the type of procedure and the speed with which your body heals this may be anything from a fortnight to several months. A slow start to the resumption of love-making is usually the best approach, with genital touching and gentle penetration later. If you have any concerns, wait until the post-operative check-up to get the all clear.

Drug treatments which induce a temporary menopause (see chapter 3) may reduce a woman's interest in sex and may cause intercourse to become less pleasurable because of a decreased output of secretions in the vagina. Fatigue due to hot flushes and sleep disturbances may also reduce sexual responsiveness. Overcoming these adverse effects calls for lateral thinking as outlined above. It will not occur overnight, so a medium- to long-term approach is vital.

Treatments for excessive bleeding, such as the Pill, progestogens, NSAIDs, danazol, and GnRH agonists are a mixed bag as far as sexual function is concerned. Some, notably progestogens and GnRH agonists, can cause a marked reduction in interest in sex; while others, such as the Pill, may produce little change.

Overcoming problems of sexual function

A hysterectomy is often seen as a last resort by women who have uterine or menstrual symptoms that are making their lives, including their sex lives, a misery. Chronic pelvic pain and protracted menstrual bleeding, for example, may mean that prior to a hysterectomy a woman's sexual needs and those of her partner are not being met. This can lead to unhappiness on all sides. A great deal of hope may be vested in the prospect of an improved relationship after hysterectomy, including an improved sexual relationship. If symptoms do not resolve quickly or new symptoms appear which continue to stymie efforts to reinstate a sexual relationship, feelings of depression may mount. Existing difficulties in a relationship may became more acute with outbursts of hostility and anger an increasingly frequent event. Short-circuiting this situation is not easy, but it may be achieved if partners can bring themselves to try pleasuring activities like massage, mechanical stimulation and mutual masturbation. In this way the very important communication that occurs via all the senses, and especially touch, can be developed.

Sexual interest, indicated by sexual arousal, sexual fantasising and masturbation, becomes apparent in females and males during the early teenage years. Then, as sexual interest matures in later adolescence, most individuals develop quite specific erotic fantasies. The ability of humans to create and respond to fantasies seems to play a major role in sexual motivation and in sexual receptivity. Strong and deliberate fantasising through erotic stories, pictures, readings and films may help stimulate this interest. Such strategies may help rekindle sexual interest.

Like most species, humans work up to sexual contact with foreplay that excites both partners. Birds coo, bow and strut. Primates spend hours grooming each other. In most mammals, delicate stimulation of sensitive body parts is an important component of stimulatory activity preceding sex. Many couples find that taking the time to gently and lovingly play with the clitoris, penis, and the nipples, using the fingers, the tongue or a vibrator, can arouse intensely pleasurable sensations. If arousal takes a long time, accept this and continue the activity only as long as you are both enjoying the experience.

There is some evidence to suggest that techniques of sexual intimacy have changed in recent generations with increases in oral sex in marriage, more variation in foreplay and more experimentation with positions. Some women enjoy deep penile penetration and may achieve this by either the female-astride position, or the man-on-top position with her legs on his shoulders and pillows under her hips. Adequate vaginal lubrication is an important consideration and can be achieved using substances such as K-Y jelly or the new hormone-free Replens which lasts for several days and is not messy. Many women find that post-menopausal hormone therapy helps lubrication. This is one of many therapies discussed in detail in the next chapter.

Lifestyle considerations

Whichever treatment is planned or has occurred, women should be aware of information about regular physical activity, pelvic floor exercises, good nutrition, hormone therapy and smoking.

Regular physical activity

Regular exercise has a remarkable effect on general well-being and the health of the body. It stimulates the lungs and blood flow (aerobic exercise), has a beneficial effect on blood clot formation and blood fat levels, lowers blood pressure and reduces the likelihood of being over-weight. Brisk walking, running, swimming and cycling are all excellent choices. Recent research indicates that muscle-strengthening resistance exercises like weight training also have a favourable effect on blood fat levels.

Reassuringly for those who do not have the urge to run or swim marathons, most of the benefits for heart health occur with moderate exercise programs. You can walk for a total of six hours a week, play golf for five hours or swim for four hours to achieve the level of activity necessary to provide significant benefits for health.

Unfortunately, nearly 40% of women around the age of menopause do not get this amount of exercise, if the Melbourne Women's Midlife Health Project is any guide. A further 15% have borderline energy expenditure levels, while just under half have good or very good weekly activity levels.

A program of regular moderate physical activity is one of the first things to consider when feeling out of sorts. In general, it is best to set a manageable target, beginning slowly and increasing the level of activity progressively. Setting too high a target can be counter-productive and may send you backwards. Sticking to an exercise plan for a couple of weeks does wonders for morale and, instead of seeking excuses to avoid exercise, you may find you can't start your activity program soon enough. In working out an exercise plan, there are some important factors to consider.

- The aim is to make regular physical activity part of your life, so choose something you enjoy — something that is convenient, interesting, can be done independently and is realistically achievable.
- If you are over forty years of age or have high blood pressure, diabetes or a known heart problem, check with your doctor before you start your plan. A preliminary health check is sometimes advisable anyway, especially if you intend working up to strenuous forms of activity.
- Always warm up for at least five minutes before exercising, and cool down afterwards. Include some stretching exercises in the warm-up to reduce the risk of muscle strain.
- Never exercise if you are not feeling well. If illness interrupts your plan, resume at a lower level and build up again slowly.

- Tell your doctor about any symptoms you experience during exercise, particularly chest discomfort or undue dizziness.

Good nutrition and weight control

Your well-being is strongly influenced by what you eat and drink. Healthy eating should not be bland or restrictive, but enjoyable and satisfying. Important features of healthy eating include low levels of fat and sugar, and plenty of water, fresh fruit and vegetables. To reduce the fat content of your meals you should:

- remove visible fat from meat and poultry
- grill, steam, microwave or boil foods rather than frying them
- use minimal oil and margarine in cooking, sauces and spreads (one to two tablespoons a day)
- eat more fish (but don't fry it!)
- choose low-fat dairy products
- limit your intake of 'hidden' fat foods such as processed meats and pastries.

Lugging around too much weight is one consequence of poor nutrition and inadequate physical activity. Another is the health risks that accumulate with the weight. Obesity increases your likelihood of developing heart disease, adult-onset diabetes and life-threatening blood clots in many parts of the body including the brain. It also makes surgery more dangerous by increasing the time it takes and the risk of complications.

Pelvic floor exercises

The muscles around the pelvis are very important in supporting the bladder, urethra, vagina and rectum. Regular practice of pelvic muscle exercises can help to strengthen these muscles. The first step is to identify the correct muscles to exercise.

- To identify the muscles around the rectum, sit or stand comfortably and imagine you are trying to control diarrhoea by consciously tightening the ring of muscles around the anus (back passage). Hold this 'squeeze' for four seconds. Relax and repeat several times.
- Now go to the toilet and start passing urine. Try to stop the flow of urine in midstream. Once this is done recommence urinating until the bladder has emptied. The muscles used to stop or slow the flow of urine are the front pelvic muscles which help control the bladder.
- Some women find they can identify the correct pelvic muscles by inserting a finger into their vagina and then contracting the pelvic muscles to squeeze the finger. If there is no sensation of squeezing around the finger you may be exercising the wrong muscles.

Note that you should not bear down as if trying to pass a bowel motion as this strengthens the wrong muscles. Do not despair if you do not seem to be making progress for several days; it may take a week or more to begin to identify the muscles that need to be exercised to strengthen and tone the pelvis.

The second step, having identified the target muscles, is to repeat the following series of exercises at least four times each day. Note that they should not be done while passing urine. With practice you will find that you can do them at any time — while waiting for a bus, watching television or setting the table.

1 While sitting or standing with thighs slightly apart, contract the muscles around the rectum followed by

the front muscles around the vagina. Hold this contraction while counting to five slowly. Relax these muscles then repeat four more times. Try to be aware of the squeezing and lifting sensation in the pelvis that occurs when these exercises are done correctly.

2 While sitting or standing, tighten the muscles around the front and back passage together. Hold this contraction for just one second and relax. Repeat this exercise five times in quick succession.

It is a good idea to return to the first step once every week or so, to check that you are using the correct muscles.

Hormone therapy

Women who have had hysterectomies or who are on certain drugs to control endometriosis are more likely than average to be prescribed hormone therapy (sometimes referred to as hormone replacement therapy or HRT). The following points should be taken into account when making a decision about whether hormone therapy is suitable for you.

- Oestrogen is effective in relieving hot flushes and night sweats, vaginal dryness and some urinary symptoms.
- Hormone therapy is particularly helpful to women who have had a premature menopause, whether it has been natural, or medically or surgically induced. They are likely to benefit most from it because they tend to suffer more extreme symptoms of menopause and are at an increased risk of osteoporosis and diseases of the heart and blood vessels, and because in many cases they no longer have a uterus and so the hormone therapy tends to be simpler (oestrogen only is usually

prescribed, but sometimes progestogen or testosterone are added).

- There is some evidence that oestrogen used on its own may offer protection against heart and blood vessel disease. This benefit is heightened for women who have had an early menopause.

- The decision about which hormone preparation is suitable for women who have not had a hysterectomy depends on the balance between several potential benefits and hazards. There are gaps in information on both sides that research will start to fill during the rest of this decade.

- In deciding whether to undertake hormone therapy for prolonged periods in the absence of worrisome symptoms, women should take account of both the anticipated benefits and the possible risks. One of the benefits of oestrogen use is that it postpones bone thinning and reduces the likelihood of heart disease. When combined with a progestogen, there are still significant benefits for bones, but progestogen appears to negate some of the protective effect that oestrogen has on the heart and blood vessel system.

- In regard to the risks, the biggest concerns lie with cancers of the breast and endometrium. Breast cancer is the most common cancer of the reproductive organs and the one most feared by women, so consideration of the link between oestrogen and breast cancer is sometimes tremendously important in helping women decide about hormone therapy. If, for a particular woman, the avoidance of an increased cancer risk is more important than the benefit in terms of osteoporosis or cardiovascular disease, this is clearly the basis on which her treatment should be decided. In making a decision, it is important that women take account of their family history of breast cancer, strokes, heart disease and osteoporosis and that they try to identify the cause of death of all close female relatives.

For many women, drawbacks to combined oestrogen and progestogen include withdrawal bleeding, break-through bleeding and PMS-like side-effects, and the possibility that hormone therapy may increase the risk of breast cancer, especially in women with a family history of this cancer.

- For women who use oestrogen on its own and who still have a uterus, an important consideration is the need for regular and extended monitoring to detect any early changes suggestive of cancer of the uterus.

Smoking

Smoking endangers heart health, as well as having a detrimental effect on our bones. If you are a twenty-cigarette-a-day smoker, you will suffer more from atherosclerosis (narrowing and plugging of arteries) than comparable non-smokers. You also have double or triple the risk of sustaining a crippling or fatal heart attack than someone of the same age, family history and activity level who does not smoke. Giving up smoking effects a rapid improvement in the health of the heart. Twelve months after quitting your risk of sudden death from heart attack is almost half that of persistent smokers and, after five years, this risk is almost identical to that of non-smokers.

Dangerous blood clots (thrombosis), which may lodge in any part of the body, can occur after surgery. Risk factors for thrombosis include being overweight and heavy smoking. If a hysterectomy, myomectomy, or endometrial resection is not urgent, it should be deferred in women who are overweight and who smoke until they have taken off excess kilos and quit smoking.

Surgeons can also help prevent thrombosis during major surgery, such as hysterectomy, by artificially stimulating the calf muscles to contract during the operation. This does no harm. Another technique is to inject an anticoagulant, such as heparin, to reduce the clotting activity of the blood. This has the disadvantage of increasing the amount of bleeding that occurs during surgery, but is generally considered preferable to the formation of a blood clot.

Women having any form of surgery should be able to recognise the early signs of thrombosis in the legs or a blood clot (embolus) in the lungs. The middle of the calf may become tender at rest or sore when moved, or the ankle may swell. An embolus in the lung may cause pain on breathing, a dry cough, shortness of breath, and soreness or pain in the chest. If any of these symptoms occur, it is important to tell your doctor or nurse promptly. An early diagnosis nearly always averts further problems.

Paradoxically, there is some evidence to suggest that women who smoke are less likely to have a hysterectomy. The reasons for this are unclear but it may be related to the suppression of oestrogen by some of the toxic components of cigarette smoke. It is presumed that smoking keeps the oestrogen required for fibroid growth under control.

eight

Questions often asked

Why have my periods become less regular, longer and heavier? I am forty-three and am in good health.

Less regular periods at forty-three years of age may be a sign of early changes in the function of your ovaries. This is a normal stage on the way to menopause when you will stop menstruating altogether. Longer and heavier periods have many causes including fibroids, endometriosis, prolapse, hormone imbalance and, rarely, cancer.

Severe premenstrual symptoms affect me for about ten days each month. Will a hysterectomy help?

Hysterectomy may help to reduce some premenstrual symptoms you may be experiencing, particularly pain, feelings of fullness in the abdomen and fatigue. It is, however, unlikely to help some other common premenstrual symptoms such as breast soreness, fluid retention, irritability or depression.

What is a Wertheim's hysterectomy?

This is another name for a radical hysterectomy, which entails the removal of the entire uterus including cervix and support structures, both ovaries, Fallopian tubes, nearby lymph nodes, and the upper portion of the vagina. It is usually performed to remove a cancer of the uterus or cervix.

What is the cause of prolapse and what treatments are effective?

Prolapse occurs when the ligaments that support the pelvic organs are damaged. This may happen during childbirth or there may be an inborn weakness of the pelvic support tissue that worsens as a normal part of the ageing process. Treatments for prolapse that have been shown to be effective in some women include hormone therapy, pelvic floor exercises, vaginal support pessaries and surgery. Of these treatments, the available evidence suggests that surgery is the most effective. It would be preferable, however, if greater emphasis was put on prevention of prolapse problems. This could be achieved by educating young women about the value of pelvic floor exercises and teaching them how to do them (see chapter 7). Ideally these exercises should be performed regularly from the teenage or early adult years onwards.

What are the different types of fibroids and how are they removed?

Fibroids may be described as subserous, intramural or submucous depending on where they are situated in the uterus. The site of the fibroid is an important consideration when deciding how it will be removed.

Subserous fibroids protrude from the outer surface of the uterus, intramural fibroids are buried in the wall of the uterus, and submucous fibroids protrude from the endometrial lining into the interior of the uterus. A further term used to describe fibroids is pedunculated. Pedunculated fibroids, usually of the subserous or submucous variety, grow at the end of a stalk.

When myomectomy is chosen as the treatment method for fibroids, the abdominal approach to entering the uterus is chosen if the fibroid is subserous or intramural. (The abdominal approach may be open cut or by laparoscopy.) If the fibroid is submucous or pedunculated submucous and the surgeon is sufficiently skilled, a hysteroscopic myomectomy may be carried out.

Fluid is sometimes used in the pelvis before a hysteroscopy to separate the abdominal organs. Could you explain why fluid is used instead of gas and the reasons why one or the other may be used? Do they have any adverse effects?

The procedure of hysteroscopy (see chapter 3) can be used for diagnosis or treatment, but in either case the uterus must be filled with something so that there is space for the hysteroscope to move about. The materials most commonly used to achieve this are carbon dioxide gas, or fluids such as glycine, dextrose, sorbitol/mannitol, saline and dextran.

Carbon dioxide has been found to be particularly useful for diagnostic hysteroscopy, but it has limited usefulness during surgery because blood causes the formation of bubbles that obscure the view. Consequently carbon dioxide gas tends to be reserved for diagnosing the cause of a problem, while fluid is the norm when hysteroscopic surgery is performed.

Occasionally the fluid or the gas is absorbed into the bloodstream, causing significant problems including an electrical imbalance of the body fluids, fluid overload, or swelling in the lungs or brain. There are several effective methods to prevent complications associated with the absorption of gas or fluid, the most important of which is for the medical team to keep a meticulous record of the amount of material instilled in the uterus and recovered from it.

I have endometriosis but it is not causing any problems at the moment. Is there any reason why I should consider having it treated?

Yes, you should consider having your endometriosis treated rather than letting it progress, as it tends to worsen in most women without treatment. Once it has progressed, it is more difficult to treat by surgery or drugs. There is, however, one circumstance in which it may be safe to ignore this advice — if your endometriosis is mild and is known not to have progressed for some years. In these circumstances, regular check-ups with ultrasound assessment are advisable.

My gynaecologist advises a hysterectomy because my fibroids have grown since I started on hormone therapy fourteen months ago. What should I do?

Fibroids only need to be treated if they are causing symptoms such as heavy or painful periods, abdominal pain, or difficulty with bowel or bladder function. Treatment is also necessary if there is any suspicion that a fibroid is turning into cancer, as indicated by its rapid growth. This is a rare occurrence, affecting only about one woman in every 800 with fibroids. If your fibroids are growing but are not causing any of the symptoms mentioned or are not suspected of becoming cancerous, then treatment is not necessary. If you are nevertheless concerned about their growth, you should consider whether you can do without hormone therapy or whether an alternative type of hormone therapy is worth trying.

Who should I see about heavy and prolonged bleeding around the time of menopause?

It would be a good idea to see a gynaecologist as heavy and prolonged bleeding near the time of menopause may be due to cancer. This possibility must be excluded before you embark on treatments such as drug therapy, endometrial resection or hysterectomy.

My sex life has deteriorated since having a hysterectomy a year ago, partly because I find it difficult to get interested in sex. I don't feel comfortable talking to my surgeon about this and I'm wondering who else could help.

Loss of interest in sex after hysterectomy may be due to reduced levels of sex hormones. This may, for example, result in less lubrication of the vagina making intercourse more painful for you. Loss of libido may also be due to feelings of depression caused by anxiety at losing the uterus and exhaustion due to the combined stresses of the condition for which you had the hysterectomy, the operation itself and the associated anaesthetic. Coincidental factors , such as relationship problems with a partner, reduced self-esteem or sexual difficulties that are unrelated to hormone levels, may be another source of difficulty. For instance, you and your partner may have drifted into a pattern of having sex which does not please you and which you are now rejecting, or your partner may have a medical condition which is making the achievement of erection more difficult for him. A general practitioner, endocrinologist, gynaecologist, psychiatrist or sex therapist may be able to help. Your doctor should be able to sort out who is best situated to provide this help, even if he or she cannot diagnose the cause of your problem.

Will I still menstruate after a hysterectomy?

No, menstruation will no longer occur. Whatever sort of hysterectomy you have will necessarily result in removal of the uterus complete with its inner lining, the endometrium, which is responsible for menstruation.

Do I really need a hysterectomy?

If you are uncertain you should seek a second opinion by consulting another specialist or asking your general practitioner for advice and for another referral. Don't be steamrolled into making a decision. It is extremely important that you are satisfied you have all the necessary information and expert advice needed before proceeding.

I am thinking about having a hysterectomy but I also need to work. How long will it take me to recover?

Your recovery time is influenced by many factors. The type of hysterectomy you have being the most important. In general, women who have a vaginal or laparoscopic hysterectomy can return to work after three to four weeks. It usually takes about two weeks longer to recover from an abdominal hysterectomy.

Other important influences on time to recovery are general fitness and weight. The fitter a woman is, the quicker her recovery, while the more overweight she is, the longer the recuperation time. Women who exercise regularly and are not overweight before hysterectomy tend to recover faster. A plan of regular exercise also helps after the operation and can commence within a few days of a vaginal or laparoscopic hysterectomy and two weeks after an abdominal hysterectomy. (The extra time is needed for wound repair.) Some women fear that activity will harm them or undo their surgery; but in virtually all gynaecological procedures, except prolapse operations, physical activity speeds recovery.

Will I put on weight after a hysterectomy?

Only if you eat as much while you are resting as you did before your operation. You should try to reduce your food intake so that it corresponds to your activity level. Boredom after surgery may result in increased eating and deleterious weight gain.

What happens to the space occupied by my uterus?

Women often wonder if an empty space remains after a hysterectomy, but you can be sure this does not occur. Organs such as the bladder, bowel and intestine reposition themselves and take up the space.

I have heard that some women get depressed after a hysterectomy. How likely is this to happen?

Recent studies suggest that, overall, rates of depression in women who have a hysterectomy are less than they were in the same women before they had the operation. In individual cases, however, depression may be increased due to complications of the operation or regrets about having it. Hysterectomy can actually reduce levels of depression in women for whom the operation relieves painful and heavy periods.

Will I age prematurely if my ovaries are removed?

The answer to this depends on whether you go on hormone therapy, your body size, whether you had your ovaries removed before or after your menopause, and your genetic make-up. Before menopause the ovaries are the body's main source of hormones such as oestrogen, which has wide-ranging influences on a woman's body. Some of the areas it affects are:
- the thickness and tone of the vaginal lining and the vagina's production of secretions
- the fullness, tone and secretions of the vulva, cervix and urethra
- bone structure and growth
- temperament and sexual interest

- the appearance and perhaps function of many other body tissues such as the skin, hair, heart, blood vessels, breasts, liver and joints.

After menopause, most women continue to make measurable and useful amounts of oestrogen in fat and muscle tissue and in the ovaries and adrenal glands (two small organs near the kidneys). How much body fat you have, and your genetic make-up, are among the most important influences on oestrogen levels after menopause.

If you have a slight build and your ovaries are removed before your menopause you are likely to experience more severe, acute menopausal symptoms (such as hot flushes, vaginal dryness, and bladder problems) than if you are well-built and you lose your ovaries after menopause. If you are in the former group, you may also find that your hair seems drier and your skin has less tone and you will also be at increased risk of heart disease and bone thinning (osteoporosis) in later life. For all these reasons you should consider oestrogen replacement therapy (a form of hormone therapy).

Women who are well-built and whose ovaries are removed before menopause tend to experience an intermediate level of symptoms and a slight to moderate increase in their long-term risk of heart disease and osteoporosis. Although such women may find oestrogen supplements useful, they may not be vitally important to their well-being.

How can I improve my health before having a hysterectomy?

Avoid smoking, have regular physical activity, and keep your weight under control. Doing these things reduces the risks associated with surgery and post-operative complications. If you are having heavy bleeds, you should take iron supplements to increase your haemo-globin level.

Will I have an early menopause if I have a hysterectomy but keep my ovaries?

In theory, removal of the uterus and cervix, but not the ovaries, should not produce menopause. The only change should be an end to your periods and removal of the problems that made the surgery necessary.

In practice, however, a significant number of women whose ovaries remain after this sort of hysterectomy do experience symptoms of menopause up to four years earlier than might be expected. Possible explanations are that the surgery inadvertently altered the blood supply to your ovaries, or the condition that caused you to have a hysterectomy in the first place, such as endometriosis or cysts, had already reduced the natural life of your ovaries.

Can you tell me about autologous blood transfusion in the lead-up to a hysterectomy?

Autologous blood transfusion is the transfusion of an individual's own blood during a surgical procedure. The blood is collected prior to surgery, a procedure that can be organised through a blood transfusion service or a hospital.

Autologous blood transfusion is usually suggested if a radical hysterectomy is proposed. This means that the surgeon intends removing the entire uterus, both ovaries, the Fallopian tubes, nearby lymph nodes and the upper portion of the vagina. However some surgeons recommend it 'just in case' for less major versions of the procedure. The amount of blood collected depends on the patient's weight and general health. If three units of blood is to be collected (a unit is 450 ml), this is done one unit at a time on three separate occasions, usually at weekly intervals. Iron supplements are usually advisable and will be prescribed by your doctor.

How much danger is involved in having a hysterectomy?

The risk to life is small — between one in 2000 and one in 5000 women who have a hysterectomy die as a result of it. The risk varies depending on the technique used, the skill of the surgical team and the reason for the hysterectomy. This is comparable to the risk of death for some other kinds of major surgery. Infection occurs after surgery in about one in twenty women, and about one in 300 sustains damage to the bladder, bowel or ureter. About one in ten women bleed after the operation. In most cases this is mild, but about one in 100 requires a blood transfusion and drainage of blood from the abdomen.

How long will I need to be in hospital?

This varies from three to seven days and may be extended by a couple of days if complications occur.

Why are antibiotics necessary?

Doctors in countries such as Australia routinely prescribe antibiotics after surgery to reduce the risk of post-operative infection.

Why am I having bowel pain after my hysterectomy?

Many women experience significant bowel pain two to four days after a hysterectomy. The sensation and the site of the pain is different from that occurring in the first day or two after surgery. The cause of the pain is temporary paralysis of the bowel which leads to constriction or swelling. As it recovers and tries to eliminate the accumulated gas and waste materials, it contracts more violently than usual.

I am still having a discharge three weeks after a hysterectomy. What is the cause of the discharge and when will it stop?

The discharge may be the result of vaginal wound healing, a wound infection, or a vaginal infection such as thrush. It usually stops one to four weeks after surgery. Occasionally it continues for a longer period of time and if this applies to you, see your doctor.

Why am I so tired since my operation?

Most people who have major surgery feel very tired in the first few weeks afterwards. This is related to the stress of the medical condition for which they had the surgery, the anxiety associated with having an operation, and the demands of surgery, anaesthesia, drugs and any postoperative complications such as anaemia or infection. If the tiredness persists for two to three months, it may be associated with a depressive reaction to the surgery. In such situations, a visit to a caring doctor is in order. Make a long appointment so that you can discuss the problem fully. If tiredness persists, it may be due to depleted oestrogen levels caused by damage to, or removal of, the ovaries at the time of the hysterectomy.

Will I need help when I come home? What about driving?

Many women find they need help with cooking and showering during the first week home. If there is no one to whom you can turn for such assistance, home help can usually be arranged through local councils with the aid of a doctor's certificate. Driving is best avoided until you are fit enough to walk up stairs and move your body freely, which usually takes two to four weeks from the time of surgery.

I had a hysterectomy three weeks ago and still find I need to take painkillers. Is this usual?

No, this sounds like there may be a problem whose diagnosis requires a medical check-up. Most healing takes place during the first two weeks after surgery so pain should have disappeared by this stage. Prolonged pain suggests there may be something amiss with the wound such as an infection, or an internal problem such as bleeding, blood clot formation, infection or adhesion formation.

When I come home after a myomectomy or hysterectomy, what will I be able to do?

Most women find that they need to rest during the first week at home, gradually increasing their activities after this. Most doctors can provide examples of abdominal exercises which can help strengthen the abdomen and improve the flexibility of the scar once the wound heals (seven to ten days). Walking or light gardening is usually possible three to six weeks after surgery. Lifting will do no harm at this stage and a gradual increase in the weight and the amount of stretching involved is beneficial. Make sure that you bend your knees and keep your back upright when lifting objects. The common worry that activities such as lifting or stretching (for example to hang washing on a clothes-line) may weaken wounds or undo stitches is groundless.

How long should I wait before resuming walking and tennis after having a hysterectomy?

Most women who have had a laparoscopic or vaginal hysterectomy can walk short distances within a week and longer distances after about three weeks. For abdominal hysterectomy, add a further two weeks. From then on, be guided by how you feel. By all means play tennis if this does not unduly distress or tire you.

I had a hysterectomy with removal of the uterus and cervix two years ago when I was twenty-eight. Am I still ovulating? What is happening to the eggs?

The ovaries should not be affected by removal of the uterus and cervix and so they are probably still releasing eggs. These pass into the abdomen where they quickly disintegrate. It is, however, not possible to give a categorical answer about what is happening to your ovaries. Even though they have not been removed, they may have been adversely affected by the hysterectomy, perhaps because of adhesion formation or perhaps due to some disturbance to their blood supply. Ovarian sex hormone production and release of eggs may diminish and menopause may occur four or so years earlier than expected.

If I have an endometrial resection, will I still have heavy menstrual periods?

After this procedure about 25% of women have no periods afterwards, 60% are having light or normal periods a year later, and 15% continue to have heavy bleeding. Within four years of an endometrial resection about 20% of women experience heavy bleeding again. Many of these women go on to have a hysterectomy.

Will I still be fertile after an endometrial resection or ablation?

Pregnancy is unlikely. If it occurs, however, the risk of complications will be above average.

Is there an increased risk of uterine cancer after endometrial resection or ablation?

There is no evidence of any increased risk at this stage. Follow-up studies to date have been reassuring although they have been of relatively short duration (covering a period of four to six years since the operation). In order to watch for any pattern of adverse effects and to study the outcome of treatment, consideration should be given to the establishment of a national register in Australia of women who have had an endometrial resection or ablation.

When my uterus was removed, it was found to be normal. Should I have had the operation?

Many women who have heavy and painful periods, or endometriosis, have a uterus that looks quite normal under the microscope. If a hysterectomy overcomes the problems that were causing them distress, they may well consider that they made the right decision. If, however, the operation fails to resolve their problems, it is reasonable for them to conclude that the operation was not necessary.

Are there any restrictions on physical activity after endometrial resection or ablation?

No, but strenuous exercise should be avoided until bleeding stops.

What are the limitations on physical activity after excisional surgery for endometriosis?

Once again, common sense is the key. You may exercise once any bleeding stops but if it makes you feel uncomfortable or tired, cut back on the activity until this is no longer a problem.

I had a hysterectomy in my mid-thirties and am now having hot flushes at the age of forty. Am I having an early menopause and what are the likely consequences of this?

Yes, what you describe is consistent with an early menopause. Apart from hot flushes you may have other symptoms of decreased oestrogen levels , such as night sweats, vaginal dryness leading to uncomfortable intercourse, and a generalised lack of 'zip'. Your early menopause puts you at increased risk of developing heart disease and osteoporosis.

How can I tell if I need hormone therapy after a hysterectomy?

This will be indicated by your experience of symptoms such as hot flushes, tiredness, insomnia, vaginal dryness and bladder irritability. Testing the levels of sex hormones in your blood is sometimes helpful in determining whether hormone therapy is called for.

How soon can I have sex after a hysterectomy?

Hysterectomy temporarily disrupts the sex life of couples, usually for three to eight weeks. Sex is possible once wound healing is complete, usually a few weeks after surgery. Some couples prefer to wait until the post-operative check-up which usually takes place about six weeks after surgery. The return to sexual intercourse should be gradual. Gentle penetration by the penis will test whether the scar is still tender. It is a good idea to discuss this aspect of recovery with your partner before you have the hysterectomy.

Will having a hysterectomy improve my sex life?

Some women lose interest in sex after a hysterectomy, but most find no change or an increase in their level of interest. If sex was enjoyable before surgery, it tends to remain so afterwards; if it was never much fun, a hysterectomy usually doesn't change that. The women who tend to find hysterectomy improves their sex life most are those with heavy bleeding, or endometriosis or adhesions which caused pelvic pain during sex. In general, however, hysterectomy is not a solution for sexual difficulties and sometimes it seems to make matters worse. If this occurs and is a worry to you, counselling by a general practitioner, endocrinologist, gynaecologist, psychologist, psychiatrist or sex therapist may prove helpful.

Am I likely to need hormone therapy after an endometrial resection?

No. This operation does not affect your ovaries or hormone balance.

Information and support services

Advice about the symptoms and conditions discussed in this book is available from family doctors, specialist medical practitioners and community health centres. Helpful information may also be obtained by telephoning the bodies listed below.

National organisations

Australian Medical Association
(06) 270 5400 or capital city in your State

Australian Natural Therapists Association
(08) 371 3222

Australian Traditional Medicine Society
(02) 809 6800

Natural Herbalists Association of Australia
(02) 502 2938

Royal Australian College of Obstetricians and Gynaecologists
(03) 417 1699

Australian Capital Territory

Women's Health Centre
(06) 290 2166

New South Wales

Albury–Wodonga Women's Centre
(060) 41 1977

Bankstown Women's Health Centre
(02) 790 1378

Bessie Smythe Foundation
(02) 764 488/764 485/764 4133

Blacktown Women's & Girls' Health Centre
(02) 831 2070/831 2022/831 2066

Blue Mountains Women's Health Centre
(047) 82 5133/82 5292

Caringbah Women's Health & Information Centre
(02) 525 2058

Central West Women's Health Centre, Bathurst
(063) 31 4133

Coffs Harbour Women's Health Centre
(066) 52 8111

Cumberland Women's Health Association, Parramatta
(02) 635 3794

Everywoman's, Leichhardt
(02) 569 9522/569 9266/560 4474

Gosford Women's Health Centre
(043) 24 2533/24 2251

Illawarra Women's Community Health Centre
(042) 96 7077

Immigrant Women's Health Service, Fairfield
(02) 726 4059

Leichhardt Women's Community Health Centre
(02) 560 3011/569 8420

Lismore & Districts Women's Health Centre
(066) 21 9627/21 9800

Liverpool Women's Health Centre
(02) 601 3555/822 5257

Newcastle Working Women's Centre
(049) 68 2511/68 2512/68 2975

Penrith Women's Health Centre
(047) 21 8749

Shoalhaven Women's Health Centre
(044) 21 1730

Wagga Wagga Women's Health Centre
(069) 21 3333/21 6209

Waminda, Nowra
(044) 21 7745

WILMA, Campbelltown
(046) 27 2955/27 2884/27 2876

Northern Territory

Family Planning Association, Darwin
(089) 48 0144

Family Planning Association, Katherine
(089) 73 8570

Family Planning Association, Alice Springs
(089) 53 0288

Queensland

Gladstone Women's Health Centre
(079) 72 7404

Gympie Women's Health Centre
(074) 83 6588

Hervey Bay Women's Health Centre
(071) 25 5788

Logan Women's Health Centre
(07) 808 9233

Mackay Women's Health Centre
(079) 53 1788

Rockhampton Women's Health Centre
(079) 22 6585 or (1800) 01 7382

Women's Health Centre, Brisbane
(07) 839 9988, (1800) 017 676 or (TTY) 831 5508

South Australia

Adelaide Women's Community Health Centre
(08) 267 5366

Endocrine, Bone and Menopause Centre, Norwood
(08) 364 3274

Tasmania

Hobart Women's Health Centre
(002) 31 3212

Victoria

Academy of Traditional Chinese Medicine
(03) 663 1363

Anti-Cancer Council of Victoria
(03) 279 1111

Cervical Cancer Support Group
(03) 596 4111 or (03) 534 1103

Cliveden Hill Private Hospital, East Melbourne
(03) 483 2500

Endometriosis Association and Clinic, Croydon
(03) 879 1276

Healthsharing Women
(03) 663 3544

Melton Community Health Centre
(03) 743 2022

Royal Women's Hospital Information Centre
(03) 344 2000

South-West Women's Health Service, Warrnambool
(055) 64 9582

The Women's Clinic on Richmond Hill
(03) 427 0399

Western Australia

Albany Community Health Women's Health Clinic
(098) 41 8244

Hedland Well Women's Centre, South Hedland
(091) 40 1124

Kalgoorlie Women's Health Centre
(090) 21 8266

Well Women's Clinic, Waratah, Bunbury
(097) 91 2884

Women's Health Care House, Northbridge, Perth
(09) 227 8122 or (008) 99 8399

Glossary

ablation completely removing tissue

adhesion fibrous connective tissue that may form between organs or other body parts after an operation

androgens sex hormones produced in small amounts by women (from the adrenal cortex and ovaries), and in large amounts by men (from the testes)

ascites an accumulation of fluid in the abdomen causing swelling

biopsy a small amount of living tissue cut from the body which is used for diagnostic purposes

colposcopy the use of an instrument, the colposcope, to visually inspect the vagina and cervix

cystocele a prolapse of the bladder into the vagina

diathermy use of high-frequency electrical currents to produce heat in the body

dilatation and curettage (D and C) a careful stretching of the cervix (dilatation) to enable entry of instruments (a curette) which remove the inner lining of the uterus (the endometrium)

dysmenorrhoea severe pain during menstruation

dyspareunia painful or difficult sexual intercourse (this term is used only for women)

electrocoagulation coagulation of tissues by means of an electrical current

endometrium the inner lining of the uterus which, during the reproductive years, is shed each month during menstruation

enterocele a loop of the intestine which is dropping down into the vagina

fibroids lumps of fibrous tissue that grow within the muscular wall of the uterus

haemorrhoids (piles) painful enlarged blood vessel(s) in the rectal or anal wall

hormone chemical messenger substance, such as oestrogen or progesterone, produced by various tissues and having a regulatory effect on other tissues

intramural fibroids fibroids that are buried in the wall of the uterus

laparoscopy a surgical procedure specifically designed to enable the doctor to look at the organs inside the abdomen by inserting a laparoscope (a tubular instrument with a light at one end and an eyepiece at the other) through a small incision in the abdominal wall

laparotomy a surgical procedure in which a large incision through the abdominal wall provides access to the pelvic organs

menopause strictly speaking, the cessation of menstruation, indicating that the ovaries have stopped producing eggs and the woman is no longer able to bear children

menorrhagia unusually heavy menstrual bleeding

myomectomy an operation involving the removal of fibroids embedded in the wall of the uterus

oophorectomy surgical removal of one or both ovaries

osteoporosis a condition in which the bones lose density and become more fragile

Pap smear a screening test to detect abnormal changes in the cells of the cervix

polycystic ovary an ovary studded with small sacs, usually filled with fluid and often associated with hormonal imbalance causing infrequent or heavy periods, hair growth and weight gain. Polycystic ovaries can be identified with an ultrasound scan. If treatment is needed, the use of laser or diathermy techniques during laparoscopy may remove them

polyp a growth protruding from any mucous membrane of the body; notably the inner lining of the uterus near the cervix. Usually has a long, tube-like appearance with a red tip. Hysteroscopic removal may be suggested if polyps are causing problems such as heavy bleeding or infertility

procidentia prolapse of the uterus into the vaginal opening

prolapse the falling or slipping down of an organ or body part from its normal position

rectocele protrusion of the rectum into the vagina

resection excision of a portion of an organ or other structure

salpingo-oophorectomy surgical removal of one or both Fallopian tubes and ovaries

submucous fibroids fibroids that protrude from the endometrial lining into the interior of the uterus

subserous fibroids fibroids that protrude from the outer surface of the uterus

ureter tube carrying urine from the kidneys to the bladder

vulva outer female genitalia surrounding the entrance to the vagina

Notes

one The uterus

1 A. Hampton and L. Salamonsen, 'Expression of messenger ribonucleic acid encoding matrix metalloproteinases and their tissue inhibitors is related to menstruation', *Journal of Endocrinology*, vol. 141, 1994, R1–R3.

2 L. Salamonsen et al. 'Immunolocalization of the vasoconstrictor endothelin in human endometrium during the menstrual cycle and in umbilical cord at birth', *American Journal of Obstetrics and Gynecology*, vol. 167, 1992, pp. 163–7.

3 Anon, 'Treatment of menorrhagia', *Lancet*, 15 August 1987, pp. 375–6.

4 K. Carlson et al. 'Indications for hysterectomy', *New England Journal of Medicine*, vol. 328, no. 12, 1993, pp. 856–60.
   L. Zussman et al. 'Sexual response after hysterectomy-oophorectomy: Recent studies and reconsideration of psychogenesis', *American Journal of Obstetrics and Gynecology*, vol. 40, no. 7, 1981, pp. 725–9.
   L. Dennerstein et al. *Gynaecology, Sex and Psyche*, Melbourne University Press, Melbourne, 1978.

V. Hufnagel, *No More Hysterectomies*, The New American Library, New York, 1988, p. 42.

5   P. E. Schwartz, 'The role of prophylactic oophorectomy in the avoidance of ovarian cancer', *International Journal of Gynaecology and Obstetrics*, vol. 39, 1992, p. 180.

6   B. S. Centerwell, 'Premenopausal hysterectomy and cardiovascular disease', *American Journal of Obstetrics and Gynecology*, vol. 139, 1981, pp. 58–61.

7   K-T. Khaw (ed.), *British Medical Bulletin Expert Review of Hormone Replacement Therapy*, vol. 48, no. 2, 1992.

8   E. Farrell and A. Westmore, *The HRT Handbook*, Anne O'Donovan, Melbourne, 1993.

9   L. Dennerstein et al. 'Hysterectomy experience amongst mid-aged Australian women', *Medical Journal of Australia*, vol. 161, 1994, pp. 311–13.

10 *For a review of these studies see* L. Dennerstein et al. *Psychosocial and Mental Health Aspects of Women's Health*, Monograph 1, World Health Organisation, Geneva, 1993. US Congress, Office of Technology Assessment, *The Menopause, Hormone Therapy, and Women's Health*, OTA-BP-BA-88, US Government Printing Office, Washington DC, May 1992, p. 23.

11 US Congress, Office of Technology Assessment, *The Menopause, Hormone Therapy, and Women's Health*, p. 22.

two Why women consider a hysterectomy

1   N. Hirsch, *Technologies for the Treatment of Menorrhagia and Uterine Myomas*, Australian

Institute of Health and Welfare HealthCare Technology Series, Canberra, no. 10, 1993, p. 1.

2 K. Carlson et al. 'Indications for Hysterectomy', *New England Journal of Medicine*, vol. 328, no. 12, 1993, pp. 856–60.

3 N. Hirsch, *Technologies for the Treatment of Menorrhagia and Uterine Myomas*, pp. 6–7.

4 I. Fraser et al. 'A preliminary study of factors influencing perception of menstrual blood loss volume', *American Journal of Obstetrics and Gynecology*, vol. 149, 1984, pp. 788–93.

5 K. Carlson et al. 'Indications for Hysterectomy', p. 858.

6 R. Shaw, 'Endometriosis — some unanswered questions', *Advances in Obstetrics and Gynaecology*, Zeneca Pharma, no. 7, 1993, p. 11.
   Anon, 'LHRH analogues in endometriosis', *Lancet*, 1 November 1986, pp. 1016–18.

7 L. Dennerstein et al. *Psychosocial and Mental Health Aspects of Women's Health*, Monograph 1, World Health Organisation, Geneva, 1993.

three Alternatives to hysterectomy

1 I. Fraser, 'Prostaglandins, prostaglandin inhibitors and menstrual disorders. Part II: Menorrhagia and premenstrual syndrome', *Healthright*, vol. 8, 1988, pp. 31–5.

2 J. Helms, 'Acupuncture for the management of primary dysmenorrhea', *Obstetrics and Gynecology*, vol. 69, no. 1, pp. 51–5.

3 C. Morse et al. 'A comparison of hormone therapy, coping skills training, and relaxation for the relief of premenstrual syndrome', *Journal of Behavioural Medicine*, vol. 14, no. 5, 1991, pp. 469–89.

4   Anon, 'Complementary medicine: A popular adjunct', *Montage* (Monash University, Melbourne), vol. 4, no. 5, 1994, p. 15.

5   K. Bone, '*Vitex agnus castus*: Scientific studies and clinical applications', *Mediherb Newsletter*, no. 42, 1994, p. 1.

6   H. K. Beecher, 'The powerful placebo', *Journal of the American Medical Association*, vol. 159, no. 17, 1955, pp. 1602–6.

7   K. Carlson et al. 'The Maine Women's Health Study. II: Outcomes of nonsurgical management of leiomyomas, abnormal bleeding, and chronic pelvic pain', *Obstetrics and Gynecology*, vol. 83, 1994, pp. 566–72.

8   K. Carlson et al. 'The Maine Women's Health Study. I: Outcomes of hysterectomy', *Obstetrics and Gynecology*, vol. 83, 1994, pp. 556–65.

9   A. Gillespie and A. Nichols, 'The value of hysteroscopy', *Australian and New Zealand Journal of Obstetrics and Gynaecology*, vol. 34, no. 1, 1994, pp. 85–7.

10 J. A. M. Broadbent et al. 'Life table analysis of treatment failure in the first four years after endometrial resection', *Gynaecological Endoscopy*, vol. 3, 1993, p. 23.

11 R. Macdonald et al. 'Endometrial ablation — a safe procedure', *Gynaecological Endoscopy*, vol. 1, 1992, pp. 7–9.

12 N. Hirsch, *Technologies for the Treatment of Menorrhagia and Uterine Myomas*, Australian Institute of Health and Welfare HealthCare Technology Series, Canberra, no. 10, 1993, p. 1.

13 C. Read, 'Trial and error in the operating theatre', *New Scientist*, 7 November 1992, pp. 12–13.

14 N. Hirsch, *Technologies for the Treatment of Menorrhagia and Uterine Myomas*, p. 31.

four Hysterectomy procedures

1   N. Hirsch, *Technologies for the Treatment of Menorrhagia and Uterine Myomas*, Australian Institute of Health and Welfare HealthCare Technology Series, Canberra, no. 10, 1993, p. 12.

2   K. Carlson et al. 'The Maine Women's Health Study. I: Outcomes of hysterectomy', *Obstetrics and Gynecology*, vol. 83, 1994, pp. 556–65.

3   K. Carlson et al. ' The Maine Women's Health Study. II: Outcomes of nonsurgical management of leiomyomas, abnormal bleeding, and chronic pelvic pain', *Obstetrics and Gynecology*, vol. 83, 1994, pp. 566–72.

4   M. J. Schofield et al. 'Self-reported long-term outcomes of hysterectomy', *British Journal of Obstetrics and Gynaecology*, vol. 98, 1991, pp. 1129–36.

5   L. Opit and D. Gadiel, *Hysterectomy in New South Wales*, Office of Health Care Finance, Sydney, 1982.

6   N. Dwyer et al. 'Randomised controlled trial comparing endometrial resection and abdominal hysterectomy for the surgical treatment of menorrhagia', *British Journal of Obstetrics and Gynaecology*, vol. 100, 1993, pp. 237–43.

7   C. de Costa, 'Hysterectomy', *Medical Journal of Australia*, vol. 157, 1992, p. 707.

8   N. Hirsch, *Technologies for the treatment of Menorrhagia and Uterine Myomas*, pp. 10–14.

9   L. Dennerstein et al. 'Hysterectomy experience amongst mid-aged Australian women', *Medical Journal of Australia*, vol. 161, 1994, pp. 311–13.

10   M. J. Sculpher et al. ' An economic evaluation of
     transcervical endometrial resection versus
     abdominal hysterectomy for the treatment of
     menorrhagia', *British Journal of Obstetrics and
     Gynaecology*, vol. 100, 1993, pp. 244–52.

five Making the treatment decision

1   C. de Costa, 'Hysterectomy', *Medical Journal of
     Australia*, vol. 157, 1992, pp. 707–8.
2   US Congress, Office of Technology Assessment, *The
     Menopause, Hormone Therapy, and Women's Health*,
     OTA-BP-BA-88, US Government Printing Office,
     Washington DC, May 1992, pp. 37–8, 49.
3   L. Dennerstein et al. *Gynaecology, Sex and Psyche*,
     Melbourne University Press, Melbourne, 1978.
     L. Opit and D. Gadiel, *Hysterectomy in New South
     Wales*, Office of Health Care Finance, Sydney, 1982.
     M. J. Schofield et al. 'Prevalence and characteristics
     of women who have had a hysterectomy in a
     community survey', *Australian and New Zealand
     Journal of Obstetrics and Gynaecology*, vol. 31, no. 2,
     1991, pp. 153–8.
     T. Selwood and C. Wood, 'Incidence of
     hysterectomy in Australia', *Medical Journal of
     Australia*, vol. 2, 1978, pp. 201–4.
4   K. Kjerulff et al. 'The socioeconomic correlates of
     hysterectomies in the United States', *American
     Journal of Public Health*, vol. 83, no. 1, 1993,
     pp. 106–8.
     M. J. Schofield et al. 'Prevalence and characteristics
     of women who have had a hysterectomy in a
     community survey'.
     L. Dennerstein et al. 'Hysterectomy experience
     amongst mid-aged Australian women', *Medical
     Journal of Australia*, vol. 161, 1994, pp. 311–13.

5   K. Carlson et al. 'The Maine Women's Health Study.
    II: Outcomes of nonsurgical management of
    leiomyomas, abnormal bleeding, and chronic pelvic
    pain', *Obstetrics and Gynecology*, vol. 83, 1994,
    pp. 566–72.

6   J. Bunker and B. Brown, 'The physician–patient as
    an informed consumer of surgical services', *New
    England Journal of Medicine*, vol. 290, no. 19, 1974,
    pp. 1051–5.

7   K. Carlson et al. 'The Maine Women's Health Study.
    I: Outcomes of hysterectomy', *Obstetrics and
    Gynecology*, vol. 83, 1994, pp. 556–65.
    K. Carlson et al. 'The Maine Women's Health Study.
    II: Outcomes of nonsurgical management of
    leiomyomas, abnormal bleeding, and chronic pelvic
    pain'.

8   A. MacLennan et al. 'The prevalence of
    hysterectomy in South Australia', *Medical Journal of
    Australia*, vol. 158, 1993, pp. 807–9.

9   T. Selwood and C. Wood, 'Incidence of
    hysterectomy in Australia'.

10 N. Hirsch, *Technologies for the Treatment of
    Menorrhagia and Uterine Myomas*, Australian
    Institute of Health and Welfare HealthCare
    Technology Series, Canberra, no. 10, 1993, p. 6.

11 A. MacLennan et al. 'The prevalence of
    hysterectomy in South Australia'.
    M. J. Schofield et al. 'Prevalence and characteristics
    of women who have had a hysterectomy in a
    community survey'.
    S. Treloar et al. 'Pathways to hysterectomy: Insights
    from longitudinal twin research', *American Journal
    of Obstetrics and Gynecology*, vol. 167, no. 1, 1992,
    pp. 82–8.

M. Ryan et al. 'Psychological aspects of hysterectomy: A prospective study', *British Journal of Psychiatry*, vol. 154, 1989, pp. 516–22.

12 L. Dennerstein et al. 'Hysterectomy experience amongst mid-aged Australian women'.

13 N. Hirsch, *Technologies for the Treatment of Menorrhagia and Uterine Myomas.*

14 L. Hancock, *Defensive Medicine and Informed Consent*, May 1993, Australian Government Publishing Service, Canberra, p. 33.

15 L. Hancock, *Defensive Medicine and Informed Consent*, p. 18.

16 Anon, 'Alternative medicine', *Choice*, October 1993, p. 8.

Bibliography

Anon. 'Alternative medicine'. *Choice*, October 1993,
pp. 7–11.

Anon. 'Complementary medicine: A popular adjunct'.
Montage, vol. 4, no. 5, 1994, p. 15.

Anon. 'Treatment of menorrhagia'. *Lancet*, 15 August
1987, pp. 375–6.

Bone, K. '*Vitex agnus castus*: Scientific studies and
clinical applications'. *Mediherb Newsletter*, no. 42,
1994, p. 1.

Broadbent, J. A. M. et al. 'Life table analysis of
treatment failure in the first four years after
endometrial resection'. *Gynaecological Endoscopy*,
vol. 3, 1993, p. 23.

Bunker, J. and Brown, B. 'The physician–patient as an
informed consumer of surgical services', *New England
Journal of Medicine*, vol. 290, no. 19, 1974,
pp. 1051–5.

Carlson, K. et al. 'Indications for hysterectomy'. *New
England Journal of Medicine*, vol. 328, no. 12, 1993,
pp. 856–60.

Carlson, K. et al. 'The Maine Women's Health Study.
I: Outcomes of hysterectomy'. *Obstetrics and
Gynecology*, vol. 83, 1994, pp. 556–65.

Carlson, K. et al. 'The Maine Women's Health Study. II: Outcomes of nonsurgical management of leiomyomas, abnormal bleeding, and chronic pelvic pain'. *Obstetrics and Gynecology*, vol. 83, 1994, pp. 566–72.

Centerwell, B. S. 'Premenopausal hysterectomy and cardiovascular disease'. *American Journal of Obstetrics and Gynecology*, vol. 139, 1981, pp. 58–61.

de Costa, C. 'Hysterectomy'. *Medical Journal of Australia*, vol. 157, 1992, pp. 707–8.

Dennerstein, L. et al. *Gynaecology, Sex and Psyche.* Melbourne University Press, Melbourne, 1978.

Dennerstein, L. et al. 'Hysterectomy experience amongst mid-aged Australian women'. *Medical Journal of Australia*, vol. 161, 1994, pp. 311–13.

Dennerstein, L. et al. *Psychosocial and Mental Health Aspects of Women's Health.* Monograph 1. World Health Organisation, Geneva, 1993.

Dwyer, N. et al. 'Randomised controlled trial comparing endometrial resection and abdominal hysterectomy for the surgical treatment of menorrhagia'. *British Journal of Obstetrics and Gynaecology*, vol. 100, 1993, pp. 237–43.

Farrell, E. and Westmore, A. *The HRT Handbook.* Anne O'Donovan, Melbourne, 1993.

Fraser, I. 'Prostaglandins, prostaglandin inhibitors and menstrual disorders. Part II: Menorrhagia and premenstrual syndrome'. *Healthright*, vol. 8, 1988, pp. 31–5.

Fraser, I. et al. 'A preliminary study of factors influencing perception of menstrual blood loss volume'. *American Journal of Gynecology and Obstetrics*, vol. 149, 1984, pp. 788–93.

Gillespie, A. and Nichols, A. 'The value of hysteroscopy'. *Australian and New Zealand Journal of Obstetrics and Gynaecology*, vol. 34, no. 1, 1994, p. 85–7.

Hampton, A. and Salamonsen, L. 'Expression of messenger ribonucleic acid encoding matrix metalloproteinases and their tissue inhibitors is related to menstruation'. *Journal of Endocrinology*, vol. 141, 1994, R1–R3.

Hancock, L. *Defensive Medicine and Informed Consent.* Australian Government Publishing Service, Canberra, May 1993.

Helms, J. 'Acupuncture for the management of primary dysmenorrhea'. *Obstetrics and Gynecology*, vol. 69, no. 1, pp. 51–5.

Hirsch, N. *Technologies for the Treatment of Menorrhagia and Uterine Myomas.* Australian Institute of Health and Welfare HealthCare Technology Series, no. 10, 1993.

Hufnagel, V. *No More Hysterectomies.* The New American Library, New York, 1988.

Khaw, K-T. (ed.). *British Medical Bulletin Expert Review of Hormone Replacement Therapy*, vol. 48, no. 2, 1992.

Kjerulff, K. et al. 'The socioeconomic correlates of hysterectomies in the United States'. *American Journal of Public Health*, vol. 83, no. 1, 1993, pp. 106–8.

Macdonald, R. et al. 'Endometrial ablation — a safe procedure'. *Gynaecological Endoscopy*, vol. 1, 1992, pp. 7–9.

MacLennan, A. et al. 'The prevalence of hysterectomy in South Australia'. *Medical Journal of Australia*, vol. 158, 1993, pp. 807–9.

Morse, C. et al. 'A comparison of hormone therapy, coping skills training, and relaxation for the relief of premenstrual syndrome'. *Journal of Behavioural Medicine*, vol. 14, no. 5, 1991, pp. 469–89.

Opit, L. and Gadiel, D. *Hysterectomy in New South Wales*. Office of Health Care Finance, Sydney, 1982.

Beecher, H. K. 'The powerful placebo'. *Journal of the American Medical Association*, vol. 159, no. 17, 1955, pp. 1602–6.

Read, C. 'Trial and error in the operating theatre'. *New Scientist*, 7 November 1992, pp. 12–13.

Ryan, M. et al. 'Psychological aspects of hysterectomy: A prospective study'. *British Journal of Psychiatry*, vol. 154, 1989, pp. 516–22.

Salamonsen, L. et al. 'Immunolocalization of the vasoconstrictor endothelin in human endometrium during the menstrual cycle and in umbilical cord at birth'. *American Journal of Obstetrics and Gynecology*, vol. 167, 1992, pp. 163–7.

Schofield, M. J. et al. 'Prevalence and characteristics of women who have had a hysterectomy in a community survey'. *Australian and New Zealand Journal of Obstetrics and Gynaecology*, vol. 31, no. 2, 1991, pp. 153–8.

Schofield, M. J. et al. 'Self-reported long-term outcomes of hysterectomy'. *British Journal of Obstetrics and Gynaecology*, vol. 98, 1991, pp. 1129–36.

Schwartz, P. E. 'The role of prophylactic oophorectomy in the avoidance of ovarian cancer'. *International Journal of Gynaecology and Obstetrics*, vol. 39, 1992, p. 180.

Sculpher, M. J. et al. 'An economic evaluation of transcervical endometrial resection versus abdominal hysterectomy for the treatment of menorrhagia'. *British Journal of Obstetrics and Gynaecology*, vol. 100, 1993, pp. 244–52.

Selwood, T. and Wood, C. 'Incidence of hysterectomy in Australia'. *Medical Journal of Australia*, vol. 2, 1978, pp. 201–4.

Shaw, R. 'Endometriosis — some unanswered questions'. *Advances in Obstetrics and Gynaecology*, Zeneca Pharma, no. 7, 1993, p. 11.

Treloar, S. et al. 'Pathways to hysterectomy: Insights from longitudinal twin research'. *American Journal of Obstetrics and Gynecology*, vol. 167, no. 1, 1992, pp. 82–8.

US Congress, Office of Technology Assessment. *The Menopause, Hormone Therapy, and Women's Health.* OTA-BP-BA-88. US Government Printing Office, Washington DC, May 1992.

Zussman, L. et al. 'Sexual response after hysterectomy-oophorectomy: Recent studies and reconsideration of psychogenesis'. *American Journal of Obstetrics and Gynecology*, vol. 40, no. 7, 1981, pp. 725–9.

Further reading

Anon. 'LHRH analogues in endometriosis'. *Lancet*, 1 November 1986, pp. 1016–18.

Anon. 'Medical rights'. *Choice*, December 1993, pp. 34–7.

Bone, K. '*Vitex agnus castus*: Scientific studies'. *Mediherb Newsletter*, February 1989, p. 1.

Coney, S. and Potter, L. *Hysterectomy*. Heinemann Reed, Auckland, 1990.

Farfalla, V. C. *Hysterectomy: Whose Choice*. Random House, Milsons Point, NSW, 1990.

Hancock, L. *Compensation and Professional Indemnity in Health Care*. Interim Report, Commonwealth Department of Human Services and Health, Canberra, February 1994.

Hicks, J. '*Vitex agnus castus*: Clinical applications'. Mediherb Newsletter, February 1989, p. 2.

Itskowic, D. 'Submucous fibroids: Clinical profile and hysteroscopic management'. *Australian and New Zealand Journal of Obstetrics and Gynaecology*, vol. 33, no. 1, 1993, pp. 63–7.

Lawrence, H. *Well-being for Women*, Lothian, Melbourne, 1990.

Lloyd, P. et al,' Choosing alternative therapy: Sociodemographic characteristics and motives of

Sydney patients'. *Australian Journal of Public Health*, vol. 17, no. 2, 1993, pp. 135–43.

Luoto, R. et al. 'Hysterectomy among Finnish women: Prevalence and women's own opinions'. *Scandinavian Journal of Social Medicine*, vol. 20, no. 4, pp. 209–12.

Maher, P. et al. 'Laparoscopically assisted hysterectomy'. *The Medical Journal of Australia*, vol. 156, 1992, pp. 316–18.

Morse, C. and Dennerstein, L. 'Cognitive therapy for premenstrual syndrome' in Brush, M. G. and Goudsmit, E. M. (eds), *Functional Disorders of the Menstrual Cycle*. Wiley, New York, 1988.

Roos, N. 'Hysterectomies in one Canadian province: A new look at risks and benefits'. *American Journal of Public Health*, vol. 74, no. 1, 1984, pp. 39–45.

Siddle, N. et al. 'The effect of hysterectomy on the age at ovarian failure: Identification of a subgroup of women with premature loss of ovarian function and literature review'. *Fertility and Sterility*, vol. 47, no. 1, 1987, pp. 94–100.

Stanton, R. *Eating for Peak Performance*. Allen & Unwin, Sydney, 1988.

Verkauf, B. 'Myomectomy for fertility enhancement and preservation'. *Fertility and Sterility*, vol. 58, no. 1, 1992, pp. 1–15.

Walker, M. et al. *Psychology*. 2nd edn. John Wiley & Sons, Milton, Qld, 1994.

Witz, C. et al. 'Complications associated with the absorption of hysteroscopic fluid media'. *Fertility and Sterility*, vol. 60, no. 5, 1993, pp. 745–55.

Wood, C. 'Alternative treatment' in Gordon, Alan (ed.), *Bailliere's Clinical Obstetrics and Gynaecology, Endometrial Ablation*, vol. 9.2, 1995.

Wood, C. 'Indications for endometrial resection'. *The Medical Journal of Australia*, vol. 156, 1992, pp. 157–160.

Wood, C. et al. 'Current status of laparoscopic associated hysterectomy'. *Gynaecological Endoscopy*, vol. 3, 1994, pp. 75–84.

Wood, C. et al. 'Laparovaginal hysterectomy'. *Australian and New Zealand Journal of Obstetrics and Gynaecology*, vol. 34, no. 1, 1994, pp. 81–4.

Wood, C. et al. 'Replacement of abdominal hysterectomy by the laparo-vaginal technique — its success and limitations'. *Australian and New Zealand Journal of Obstetrics and Gynaecology*, vol. 34, no. 5, (in press).

Wood, C. et al. 'The value of vaginal ultrasound in the management of menorrhagia'. *Australian and New Zealand Journal of Obstetrics and Gynaecology*, vol. 33, no. 2, 1993, pp. 198–201.

Index